Cancer Pain Management
SCENARIOS

Edited by
Michele E. Gaguski, MSN, RN, CHPN, AOCN®, APN-C
Susan D. Bruce, RN, MSN, OCN®

Oncology Nursing Society
Pittsburgh, Pennsylvania

ONS Publishing Department
Executive Director, Professional Practice and Programs:
Elizabeth M. Wertz Evans, RN, BSN, MPM, CPHQ, CPHIMS, FHIMSS, FACMPE
Publisher and Director of Publications: Barbara Sigler, RN, MNEd
Managing Editor: Lisa M. George, BA
Technical Content Editor: Angela D. Klimaszewski, RN, MSN
Staff Editor II: Amy Nicoletti, BA
Copy Editor: Laura Pinchot, BA
Graphic Designer: Dany Sjoen

Library of Congress Cataloging-in-Publication Data
Cancer pain management scenarios / edited by Michele E. Gaguski, Susan D. Bruce.
    p. ; cm.
Includes bibliographical references.
ISBN 978-1-935864-28-8 (alk. paper)
I. Gaguski, Michele E. II. Bruce, Susan D. III. Oncology Nursing Society.
[DNLM: 1. Pain Management–nursing–Examination Questions. 2. Analgesics–therapeutic use--Examination Questions. 3. Neoplasms–complications–Examination Questions. 4. Neoplasms–nursing–Examination Questions. WY 18.2]
    RB127
    616'.0472076–dc23

                                                            2013003215

Publisher's Note
This book is published by the Oncology Nursing Society (ONS). ONS neither represents nor guarantees that the practices described herein will, if followed, ensure safe and effective patient care. The recommendations contained in this book reflect ONS's judgment regarding the state of general knowledge and practice in the field as of the date of publication. The recommendations may not be appropriate for use in all circumstances. Those who use this book should make their own determinations regarding specific safe and appropriate patient-care practices, taking into account the personnel, equipment, and practices available at the hospital or other facility at which they are located. The editors and publisher cannot be held responsible for any liability incurred as a consequence from the use or application of any of the contents of this book. Figures and tables are used as examples only. They are not meant to be all-inclusive, nor do they represent endorsement of any particular institution by ONS. Mention of specific products and opinions related to those products do not indicate or imply endorsement by ONS. Web sites mentioned are provided for information only; the hosts are responsible for their own content and availability. Unless otherwise indicated, dollar amounts reflect U.S. dollars.

ONS publications are originally published in English. Publishers wishing to translate ONS publications must contact ONS about licensing arrangements. ONS publications cannot be translated without obtaining written permission from ONS. (Individual tables and figures that are reprinted or adapted require additional permission from the original source.) Because translations from English may not always be accurate or precise, ONS disclaims any responsibility for inaccuracies in words or meaning that may occur as a result of the translation. Readers relying on precise information should check the original English version.

Printed in the United States of America

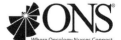

Oncology Nursing Society
Integrity • Innovation • Stewardship • Advocacy • Excellence • Inclusiveness

Contributors

Editors

Michele E. Gaguski, MSN, RN, CHPN, AOCN®, APN-C
Clinical Director
Medical Oncology/Infusion Services
AtlantiCare Cancer Care Institute
Egg Harbor Township, New Jersey

Susan D. Bruce, RN, MSN, OCN®
Oncology Clinical Nurse Specialist
Duke Raleigh Cancer Center
Raleigh, North Carolina

Field Reviewers

Maureen Lynch, MS, APRN, AOCN®, ACHPN
Nurse Practitioner, Adult Palliative Care
Dana-Farber Cancer Institute
Boston, Massachusetts

Fabienne Ulysse, DNP, ANP, AOCNP®
Assistant Professor of Nursing
Long Island University
Brooklyn, New York
Oncology Clinical Coordinator
Lutheran Medical Center
Brooklyn, New York

Julie Vosit-Steller, DNP, FNP-BC, AOCN®
Associate Professor of Practice
Simmons College School of Nursing and Health Sciences
Boston, Massachusetts
Palliative Care Consultant
Brigham and Women's Faulkner Hospital
Boston, Massachusetts

Disclosure

Editors and authors of books and guidelines provided by the Oncology Nursing Society (ONS) are expected to disclose to the readers any significant financial interest or other relationships with the manufacturer(s) of any commercial products.

A vested interest may be considered to exist if a contributor is affiliated with or has a financial interest in commercial organizations that may have a direct or indirect interest in the subject matter. A "financial interest" may include, but is not limited to, being a shareholder in the organization; being an employee of the commercial organization; serving on an organization's speakers bureau; or receiving research from the organization. An "affiliation" may be holding a position on an advisory board or some other role of benefit to the commercial organization. Vested interest statements appear in the front matter for each publication.

Contributors are expected to disclose any unlabeled or investigational use of products discussed in their content. This information is acknowledged solely for the information of the readers.

The contributors provided the following disclosure and vested interest information:

Michele E. Gaguski, MSN, RN, CHPN, AOCN®, APN-C, consultant or advisory role, ONS, CDC Advisory Board; honoraria, ONS

Susan D. Bruce, RN, MSN, OCN®, honoraria, Allos Therapeutics

Mary Pat Johnston, RN, MS, AOCN®, leadership position, ONS Board of Directors, liaison to Oncology Nursing Certification Corporation; honoraria, Amgen, Novartis, ONS

Contents

The reader is referred to Appendices A and B (pp. 91–96) to assist with answering questions related to the case studies.

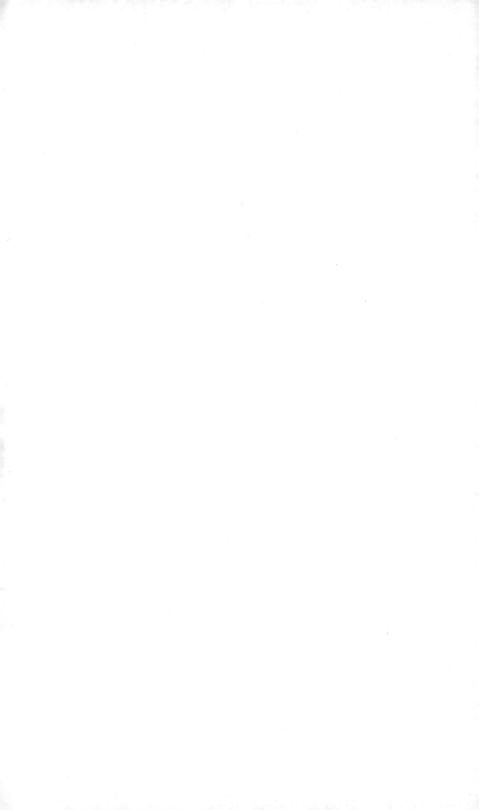

A 67-Year-Old Man With Prostate Cancer

J.S. is a 67-year-old Caucasian man who was diagnosed with stage III prostate cancer in 2009. He was initially diagnosed with a T3 (extracapsular presence of tumor), N1 (regional lymph node metastasis), M0 (no evidence of distant metastasis) tumor; therefore, evidence-based treatment included surgical treatment with a retropubic prostatectomy followed by a course of external beam radiation treatments daily for five weeks (National Cancer Institute, 2012). J.S. recovered well with the exception of urinary incontinence, which was treated with pelvic floor strengthening exercises (Kegel exercise) and urinary control products such as incontinence pads. J.S. returned to a fairly active life following surgical recovery and followed up with his oncologist every six months. On his next follow-up visit, his prostate-specific antigen (PSA) result was 1.4 ng/dl. This level indicates a possible return of prostate cancer. J.S. was scheduled for a repeat PSA and bone scan to evaluate for recurrence and to determine if further treatment is indicated.

This morning, J.S. awoke with a sharp pain in his lower back with numbness and tingling in his lower legs. These symptoms improved slightly after getting out of bed and standing. He attributed this pain to "sleeping wrong" or "overexertion yesterday," as he had a very active day that included nine holes of golf and an evening of dancing with his wife.

J.S.'s wife was troubled by his gait, which she noted was unsteady compared to the previous day. When J.S. attempted to urinate, he experienced difficulty initiating the stream and had to brace himself against the wall for balance. He reported a shooting pain that started as he walked out of the bathroom and resulted in a fall to the floor. His wife came to his aid but was unable to help him up, so she called 911.

When the emergency medical technicians arrived, they placed J.S. in a supine position on a backboard for transport to the hospital.

J.S. rated his pain as a 10 on a 0–10 numeric scale. He described the pain as shooting and feeling as if a band was around his lower back and abdomen. He also reported tingling from his back that radiated to his left buttock. His wife called the oncologist, who arranged for a direct admission to the inpatient oncology unit. You are the nurse assigned to J.S. on the oncology unit.

The oncologist orders a magnetic resonance imaging (MRI) scan and a bone scan. Based on J.S.'s symptoms, the most likely rationale for these tests is to rule out
a. Prostate cancer recurrence.
b. Sciatic pain.
c. Spinal cord compression.
d. Osteoporosis.

The correct answer is c. Based on J.S.'s symptoms of back pain, numbness and tingling, altered gait, and pain that improves when upright, spinal cord compression is the most appropriate rationale for the tests ordered. In addition, prostate cancer is associated with spinal cord compression. Approximately 5%–10% of all patients with prostate cancer will experience malignant spinal cord compression (MSCC), with higher incidence among patients whose tumors are hormone-resistant (Benjamin, 2002). Patients with prostate cancer account for 15%–20% of all MSCC cases (Abrahm, Patchell, & Rades, 2009). Answer a is incorrect because prostate cancer recurrence alone would not account for neurologic symptoms. Answer b is incorrect because sciatic back pain is usually unilateral and aggravated by movement, and J.S.'s symptoms improved when he got out of bed. Answer d is incorrect because osteoporosis is not diagnosed with MRI, and it is a symptomless disease.

J.S.'s MRI revealed bony metastasis at T-12 and S1 with a spinal cord compression. The oncologist told J.S. and his wife that he had metastatic disease and spinal cord compression.

The most common cause of cancer pain is
a. Bone metastasis.
b. Liver metastasis.
c. Pancreatic involvement.
d. Brain metastasis.
The correct answer is a. Bone metastasis is the leading cause of cancer pain (Davar & Honore, 2002).

As the nurse assessing J.S., you inquire about the location and precipitating symptoms of his pain. The usual symptoms of a suspected spinal cord compression include all of the following *except*
a. Pain that improves when lying down.
b. Pain that is localized in the back.
c. Pain that increases with sneezing.
d. Pain that increases with neck flexion.
The correct answer is a. Pain from MSCC improves when sitting or standing. This is in contrast to disc disease, which is relieved by lying down (Miaskowski et al., 2005). Answers b, c, and d describe pain symptoms common in MSCC. Pain tends to be localized at the region of cord compression and may increase with coughing, sneezing, or any increase in intrathoracic pressure, as well as with neck flexion (Hunter, 2005).

You receive several physician orders for J.S. Which order is indicated for both treatment of spinal cord compression and pain?
a. Morphine 4 mg IV push now, and then every four hours

b. Dexamethasone 96 mg IV bolus now, followed by 24 mg PO every six hours
c. Zoledronic acid 4 mg IV piggyback over 15 minutes, now
d. Lorazepam 1 mg PO now, and every six hours PRN
   The correct answer is b. Dexamethasone is a corticosteroid that works at the tissue level to lower free water content, reduce prostaglandin E_2 levels, and decrease the spinal cord–specific gravity. These three actions help to both reduce spinal cord swelling, decreasing onset of paralysis, and improve pain and neurologic functioning (Rodvelt, 2007). Answer a is incorrect because morphine is an opioid and treats the pain but does not affect the spinal cord compression. Answer c is incorrect because zoledronic acid is indicated for the treatment of bone metastasis but does not have a direct role in pain management. Answer d is incorrect because lorazepam is a benzodiazepine used to treat anxiety.

What is the most commonly used treatment for MSCC management?
a. Surgical stabilization
b. Chemotherapy
c. Surgery followed by radiation
d. Radiation therapy
   The correct answer is d. Radiation therapy is the most commonly used approach for managing MSCC. Typically, an MRI is performed to identify areas of spinal cord compression. Radiation is targeted to the site of compression and the two vertebrae above and below this site. Length of therapy is two to four weeks with a dosage range of 30–50 Gy. Radiation treatment is administered concomitantly with steroids. The steroids are tapered during the radiation treatment (Abrahm,

Banffy, & Harris, 2008). Answer a is incorrect because surgical stabilization is used for patients who have developed MSCC in sites previously treated with radiation, and in those whose symptoms worsen while receiving radiation. Answer b is incorrect because chemotherapy is not used for treatment of this condition. Answer c is incorrect because radiation would not be used following surgery to the spine.

J.S. was hospitalized for a week for symptom management, pain control, and progressive physical therapy. While on the inpatient oncology unit, he was transitioned from round-the-clock IV morphine to oral morphine. J.S.'s total dose in 24 hours was 30 mg IV.

To convert J.S.'s IV morphine dose to oral morphine, the nurse must first
a. Multiply the 24-hour IV dose of morphine by 3.
b. Divide the 24-hour IV dose of morphine by 2.
c. Use the IV dose as the equivalent for the oral dose.
d. Divide the dose of IV morphine by 12.
The correct answer is a. To convert from IV morphine to oral morphine, the practitioner must first calculate the average daily (24-hour) IV dose of morphine used. Then, use the equianalgesic conversion of a 1:3 ratio of IV to PO morphine (e.g., 10 mg IV morphine is equivalent to 30 mg PO morphine) (Mercadante, 2010; Mercadante, Villari, Ferrera, Bianchi, & Casuccio, 2004). Answer b is incorrect because dividing would provide too small a dose based on his 24-hour IV usage. Answer c is incorrect because the correct IV dose is one-third of the total oral dose. Answer d is incorrect because this is the wrong equianalgesic calculation. Therefore, J.S.'s oral dose would be 90 mg. He was started on long-acting morphine 45 mg every 12 hours.

Which of the following would be an appropriate initial bowel regimen order for J.S. to take with this opioid regimen?

a. Bisacodyl 5 mg daily and docusate sodium 100 mg twice a day
b. No bowel regimen needed
c. Milk of magnesia 30 mg every three hours
d. Cholestyramine powder 15 g three times a day

The correct answer is a. Patients taking daily round-the-clock opioids require a bowel regimen to avoid significant constipation. The opioid effect on opioid receptors in the bowel slows peristalsis. Although tolerance to other side effects may develop, tolerance to constipation will not occur. The use of stimulant laxatives and stool softeners provides effective prevention in most patients (Wong, 2007). Answer b is incorrect because a patient receiving opioids should automatically be started on a bowel regimen; this is the standard of care. Answer c is incorrect because this dosage schedule exceeds the recommended daily dose for this medication and is too frequent and inconvenient for a maintenance regimen. Answer d is incorrect because cholestyramine powder is a medication used to lower cholesterol that causes constipation.

Following discharge, J.S. completed three weeks of radiation therapy and was tapered off dexamethasone. At his next appointment, J.S.'s PSA level was elevated; therefore, he underwent a prostate biopsy that confirmed prostate cancer recurrence. Using the National Comprehensive Cancer Network (2012) guidelines for prostate cancer, J.S.'s oncologist recommended androgen deprivation therapy and ordered a three-week cycle of the antiandrogen flutamide 250 mg PO daily and monthly bisphosphonate therapy to treat the bone metastases. After the initial three-week cycle, J.S. began treatment with a luteinizing hormone-releasing hormone (LHRH). The rationale for the three-week window of strictly antiandrogen therapy is to prevent the initial flare phenomenon. This flare is thought to be caused by an initial surge of testosterone when the LHRH receptors are stimulated. This condition may be life threatening in men who have high-volume metastatic prostate cancer. Treating with antiandrogen therapy first inhibits the stimulatory effect and prevents this testosterone surge. At his next appointment with the physician, J.S. indicated his pain was much improved, he was sleeping well, and his leg weakness was almost imperceptible. He had not had any further incidents of falling and was returning to his former activity level. He denied any further urinary problems or any new symptoms.

References

Abrahm, J., Banffy, M., & Harris, M. (2008). Spinal cord compression in patients with advanced metastatic cancer: "All I care about is walking and living my life". *JAMA, 299,* 937–946. doi:10.1001/jama.299.8.937

Abrahm, J., Patchell, R., & Rades, D. (2009). Personalized treatment for malignant spinal cord compression: A multidisciplinary approach. In *2009 ASCO educational book* (pp. 555–562). Retrieved from http://www.asco.org/ASCOv2/Home/Education%20&%20Training/Educational%20Book/PDF%20Files/2009/09EdBk.PatientCare.04.pdf

Benjamin, R. (2002). Neurologic complications of prostate cancer. *American Family Physician, 65,* 1834–1841. Retrieved from http://www.aafp.org/afp/2002/0501/p1834.html

Davar, G., & Honore, P. (2002). What causes cancer pain? *Pain: Clinical Updates, 10*(2). Retrieved from http://www.iasp-pain.org/AM/AMTemplate.cfm?Section=Home&CONTENTID=7593&TEMPLATE=/CM/ContentDisplay.cfm&SECTION=Home

Hunter, J. (2005). Structural emergencies. In J.K. Itano & K.N. Taoka (Eds.), *Core curriculum for oncology nursing* (4th ed., pp. 422–442). St. Louis, MO: Elsevier Saunders.

Mercadante, S. (2010). Intravenous morphine for management of cancer pain. *Lancet Oncology, 11,* 484–489. doi:10.1016/S1470-2045(09)70350-X

Mercadante, S., Villari, P., Ferrera, P., Bianchi, M., & Casuccio, M. (2004). Safety and effectiveness of intravenous morphine for episodic (breakthrough) pain using a fixed ratio with the oral daily morphine dose. *Journal of Pain and Symptom Management, 27,* 352–359. doi:10.1016/j.jpainsymman.2003.09.006

Miaskowski, C., Cleary, J., Burney, R., Coyne, P., Finley, R., Foster, R., … Zahrbock, C. (2005). *APS Clinical Practice Guideline Series No. 3: Guideline for the management of cancer pain in adults and children.* Glenview, IL: American Pain Society.

National Cancer Institute. (2012, September 21). Prostate cancer treatment (PDQ®): Stage information for prostate cancer. Retrieved from http://www.cancer.gov/cancertopics/pdq/treatment/prostate/HealthProfessional/page3

National Comprehensive Cancer Network. (2012). *NCCN Clinical Practice Guidelines in Oncology: Prostate cancer* [v.3.2012]. Retrieved from http://www.nccn.org/professionals/physician_gls/pdf/prostate.pdf

Rodvelt, T. (2007). Management and treatment of bone disease. In R. Ignaffo, C. Viele, & Z. Ngo (Eds.), *Mosby's oncology drug reference* (pp. 391–419). St. Louis, MO: Elsevier Mosby.

Wong, P. (2007). Supportive care of the cancer patient. In R. Ignaffo, C. Viele, & Z. Ngo (Eds.), *Mosby's oncology drug reference* (pp. 421–436). St. Louis, MO: Elsevier Mosby.

Rachel Behrendt, DNP, RN, AOCN®
Vice President, Nursing Professional Development
and Magnet Recognition Program
Thomas Jefferson University Hospital
Philadelphia, Pennsylvania

A 54-Year-Old Man With Chronic Lower Back and Post-Thoracotomy Pain

S.D. is a 54-year-old construction worker with a history of chronic lower back pain. In early September he recovered from symptoms he attributed to a bad summer cold, but his cough persisted and became uncomfortable. He went to his primary care physician (PCP) and was given a course of antibiotics; however, his symptoms did not improve. He had several episodes of hemoptysis and was sent for a chest x-ray, followed by a positron-emission tomography/computed tomography scan that revealed a lesion in the right lower lobe of the lung measuring 2.6 cm × 3.1 cm. He was evaluated by a thoracic surgical oncologist and underwent a thoracotomy and a lobectomy. Tissue pathology confirmed adenocarcinoma non-small cell lung cancer, stage 1B. Before experiencing symptoms of lung cancer, S.D. was already taking 10 mg oxycodone continuous release (CR) BID and 5 mg oxycodone with acetaminophen (Percocet®) every four to six hours PRN for chronic lower back pain, ordered by his PCP. The chronic back pain was the result of a work injury and unrelated to his surgical pain issues or cancer.

Prior to surgery, S.D. rated his back pain as 3 out of 10 on the 0–10 numeric rating scale (NRS) while receiving the above listed combination of long- and short-acting opioids for chronic back pain. On initial assessment he identified his pain goal to be 3 out of 10. Immediately post thoracotomy, S.D. was prescribed hydromorphone via patient-controlled analgesic (PCA) pump. Initially, the PCA was programmed for breakthrough dosing only. He remained on the PCA with dosing added as a continuous infusion (0.2 mg per hour) and with PCA doses (0.2 mg with a lockout of 20 minutes, available for breakthrough pain). Three days after surgery, S.D. reported to his nurse that his pain was 5 out of 10 on the NRS. At this point, his nurse instructed him to continue to use his PCA for breakthrough pain and collaborated with the clinical team to achieve his pain goal of 3 out of 10.

Later that day the thoracic surgeon assessed S.D. and decided to wean him off the PCA. The surgeon stated, "With his past use of opioids, I'd feel better having him receive only oral pain medications." The right chest tube was still in place. In the progress note, the surgeon wrote that the patient appeared comfortable and he planned to immediately wean S.D. off the continuous-infusion portion of the PCA and the following day would discontinue the PCA completely. He ordered oxycodone CR 10 mg PO BID. To manage breakthrough pain, the surgeon ordered one to two tablets Percocet PO every four hours for moderate pain and hydromorphone 2 mg PO every two hours for severe pain.

Immediately after the PCA was discontinued (four days after surgery), S.D. reported pain levels of 7 out of 10. He became angry with the staff and deliberately knocked items off of his tray table. The staff nurses discussed among themselves how he "never appeared" to be in pain, that at times he was found quietly watching TV. His nurse said that whenever she entered the room he insisted his pain was 10 out of 10 and he demanded more medication. One nurse said, "I know pain is what the patient says it is, but I'm worried that he is over-exaggerating his pain."

In a few days, his behavior became so disruptive that his assigned nurse asked the charge nurse for a meeting to discuss his care. At the meeting, the charge nurse encouraged the staff to voice their concerns. Two nurses admitted that it was a challenge to assess his pain, that they found his reports of pain not believable, and that they attributed his frequency of requesting medication as a possible sign of addiction. This behavior caused the staff nurses to experience doubts about being effective in controlling his pain. One of the nurses was concerned that by giving him pain medications as often as he requested, she was contributing to an addiction. At the end of the meeting, the charge nurse reminded the staff that it is important to make a distinction between believing the report of pain and accepting it. She explained that according to Pasero and McCaffery (2011), a common reason for not believing a patient's report of pain is the fear of causing or contributing to addiction. During the meeting, the staff requested a palliative care team consult. Based on the patient's diagnosis and reports of pain, as well as the nurses' concerns about the patient's possible addictive behavior, those who attended the meeting found a consultation with the palliative care team to be an acceptable solution.

Which of the following should *not* be included in the nurse's assessment of pain?

a. Assess aggravating and alleviating factors of pain.
b. Ask the patient to describe the pain (e.g., sharp, shooting, burning).
c. Disregard the patient's report of pain on the NRS if the patient does not show any behavioral signs of pain.
d. Consider the patient's history of opioid use, which may include tolerance and the need for higher doses of pain medication to achieve adequate pain management.

The correct answer is c. Pain reports and pain behaviors may be incongruent, but an absence of pain behaviors is not proof that pain is not present. Pain should always be assessed by more than just the NRS. Nurses must accept the report of pain. Answers a, b, and d are all appropriate to include in a pain assessment. Staff should encourage each other to consider other strategies for addressing pain when a climate of suspicion develops and is affecting patient care (Pasero & McCaffery, 2011).

Addiction is defined as

a. A physiologic state characterized by a decrease in the effects of a drug after chronic administration, or by a need for a higher dose to maintain effectiveness.
b. The physiologic adaptation of the body to the presence of an opioid. Withdrawal symptoms occur when opioids are discontinued, the dose is abruptly reduced, or when an antagonist is added.
c. A neurobiologic disorder characterized by impaired use of drugs for nonmedical reasons, a craving for drugs, and continued use despite harm.

    d. Escalating demand for medication, asking for medication before the prescribed interval time, and obtaining medications from others. Behavior resolves when pain is effectively treated.

    The correct answer is c. Opioid addiction may include symptoms of tolerance or dependence, but the key features include changes in behavior, impaired control of drug use, and continued use of medication despite harm. Answer a defines tolerance, which is a normal response to regular administration of pain medication. Answer b defines physical dependence, which is a normal response that occurs with repeated administration of medications, usually more than two weeks. Answer d describes pseudo-addiction, often confused with true addiction but distinguished by a resolution of behaviors once pain is treated effectively (Pasero & McCaffery, 2011, p. 33).

    Five days after surgery, the palliative care team facilitated a family meeting, which included the patient, his sister, two staff nurses, the physician, and the charge nurse. S.D. was given the opportunity to voice his concerns regarding the management of his pain. He revealed that in addition to his pain, he was nervous and uncomfortable about being in the hospital. He thought of the hospital as a place where people go to die. A treatment plan for managing his pain was established and agreed upon by the patient and the staff. One aspect of the plan was providing continuity of nursing care. S.D. identified the nurses he had worked closely with, and the charge nurse agreed these nurses would be part of his care team. As part of the immediate plan, it was agreed that for the remainder of the day, S.D. would be offered hydromorphone PO every two hours on round-the-clock scheduling. The nurses asked S.D. if he wished to be awakened when his breakthrough medication was due, and S.D. agreed to this plan. After eight hours, the palliative care team would reassess his pain level as well as his response to the care plan.

    According to the Oncology Nursing Society (ONS, n.d.) Putting Evidence Into Practice (PEP) guidelines for pain assessment and management, when a patient continues to express the same level of pain without relief, the nurse should discuss with the physician and the palliative care team the need to increase the medication in an attempt to alleviate the pain and to consider a pain team consult. Nonpharmacologic interventions, such as use of a heating pad, distraction, or pet therapy, should be integrated with pharmacologic treatment. S.D. had enjoyed a previous visit from a pet therapy dog. The patient was offered a visit from the chaplain, but he declined. These alternative pain treatments were integrated into the pain management plan for S.D. and helped increase his sense of control over the situation (ONS, n.d.). The staff nurse provided education to S.D. and his sister regarding opioid tolerance and his need for increased medication to alleviate his pain and achieve his goals.

When the palliative care advanced practice nurse returned to assess S.D.'s pain, he reported some relief of pain, rating it 6 out of 10 compared to his previous report of 10 out of 10. He was satisfied with the progress since implementing the plan of care; he also reported feeling less nervous about being in the hospital. After the meeting, the staff debriefed with the palliative care team. The palliative care physician introduced the concept of *total pain* as defined by Dame Cicely Saunders, the founder of the modern hospice movement. The palliative care physician shared a quote made by Dame Saunders: "I coined the term 'total pain' from my understanding that dying people have physical, spiritual, psychological, and social pain that must be treated." The group discussed that although S.D. was not dying, he exhibited signs of total pain because of his diagnosis and his behavior in regard to pain medications (Field, 2012; Halifax, 2011).

Total pain includes the assessment of nonphysical aspects of pain, such as anxiety and fear. According to Dame Saunders, what are the four domains of total pain?
a. Physical, nociceptive, neuropathic, and comfort
b. Emotional, physical, transcendental, and mindfulness
c. Physical, social, spiritual, and emotional
d. Physical, psychological, spiritual, and social
   The correct answer is d. While the physical aspects of pain are often the easiest to assess, the other domains (psychological, spiritual, and social) have a significant im-

pact on the patient's perception of pain. Dame Saunders is quoted as saying, "Constant pain needs constant control" (Richmond, 2005, p. 238).

The following day, S.D. stated that he felt as if his concerns were heard and his pain needs were being sufficiently addressed. The nurses were also satisfied with implementing evidence-based care and seeing the improved outcomes. After his chest tube was removed, S.D. reported his pain as 4 out of 10, which was close to his pain goal of returning to 3 out of 10. His pain medications were eventually decreased to his preadmission dose. S.D. was instructed to resume his preadmission analgesic regimen and to follow up with the outpatient palliative care clinic and his medical oncologist one week after discharge.

References

Field, B. (2012). Science hero: Dame Cicely Saunders. Retrieved from http://www.myhero.com/go/hero.asp?hero=Cicely_Saunders_06

Halifax, J. (2011). The precious necessity of compassion. *Journal of Pain and Symptom Management, 41*, 146–153. doi:10.1016/j.painsymman.2010.08.010

Oncology Nursing Society. (n.d.). PEP: Pain. Retrieved from http://www.ons.org/Research/PEP/Pain

Pasero, C., & McCaffery, M. (2011). *Pain assessment and pharmacologic management.* St. Louis, MO: Elsevier Mosby.

Richmond, C. (2005). Dame Cicely Saunders: Founder of the modern hospice movement. *BMJ, 331*, 238. doi:10.1136/bmj.331.7510.238

Ann Brady, MSN, RN-BC
Symptom Management Care Coordinator, Oncology
Huntington Hospital Cancer Center
Pasadena, California

An 83-Year-Old Woman With Metastatic End-Stage Breast Cancer

R.S. is an 83-year-old woman with stage IV breast cancer and metastases to the ribs and right lung. Her history included a right mastectomy followed by adjuvant external beam radiation therapy, hypertension, and advanced dementia. R.S. was admitted to the hospital from a skilled nursing facility (SNF) because of increased shortness of breath. She presented with a large right pleural effusion and underwent a thoracentesis. The procedure dramatically improved her symptoms, and R.S.'s physician determined that she could be discharged within 24 hours. R.S.'s daughter indicated that she "does not want her mother to suffer" and told the medical team that the primary goal for her mother's care was comfort and symptom management. The plan was to discharge R.S. to the SNF and to provide a referral to a hospice agency. During her hospital admission, R.S. called out frequently, appeared restless, and was observed rubbing her right chest wall.

What does the nurse need to consider when evaluating R.S.'s pain status?
a. Patients with dementia experience less pain than those without dementia.
b. R.S. may have difficulty expressing her pain.
c. R.S. will require more pain medication than most patients.
d. Patients with dementia should not be asked to self-report pain.

The correct answer is b. Older adults with cognitive impairment may have difficulty expressing their pain and using traditional rating scales. Although the gold standard for pain assessment is a patient's report, patients with cognitive impairment may only be able to express their pain nonverbally, such as by moaning, grimacing, moving restlessly, or lying very still. Answers a and c are incorrect, as no evidence supports that patients with dementia experience more or less pain than patients without cognitive impairment (Coyle & Derby, 2006; Huffman & Kunik, 2000). Answer d is also incorrect. All patients should be asked to self-report their pain; however, if a patient has cognitive impairment, other methods of assessing pain and the response to interventions may be required. The Pain Assessment in Advanced Dementia (PAIN-AD) and the Assessment of Discomfort in Dementia are examples of behavioral pain assessment tools (Herr et al., 2006). According to Herr and colleagues (2006), behavioral pain scores are not comparable to standard pain intensity ratings but are helpful in assessing the response to interventions. Using a standard approach to nonverbal pain assessment provides a less subjective approach among providers; however, no single approach to pain assessment works for all patients (Herr et al., 2006).

R.S.'s nonverbal pain score was 7 out of 10 using the PAIN-AD. Her PRN medications included oxycodone 5 mg PO every eight hours for severe pain and acetaminophen 650 mg PO every six hours for moderate pain. R.S. was disoriented but able to recognize her daughter. R.S. repetitively answered "no" to all questions.

What would be the best approach to manage R.S.'s pain?
a. Offer only oxycodone for severe pain.
b. Administer acetaminophen as needed for moderate pain.
c. Alternate between doses of oxycodone and acetaminophen.
d. Consider oxycodone around the clock.

The correct answer is d. Use of regularly scheduled pain medication, starting at a low dose and slowly increasing the dose as indicated by pain assessment, would be an appropriate plan (McCaffery, Herr, & Pasero, 2011). Answer a is incorrect. Offering pain medications at regular intervals may be an effective strategy for a cognitively intact adult, but a cognitively impaired person may not be able to verbalize her need for pain medication (McCaffery et al., 2011). Answers b and c are also incorrect. According to the three-step World Health Organization Pain Relief Ladder, step 1 addresses mild pain by suggesting a nonopioid, such as acetaminophen or a nonsteroidal; step 2 is to assist the clinician in selecting the opioid that may be conventionally preferred for the treatment of moderate to severe pain in the patient who is opioid-naïve or nearly so (Pasero, Quinn, Portenoy, McCaffery, & Rizos, 2011). R.S.'s nonverbal pain rating is a 7 and requires round-the-clock dosing to attempt to manage her pain most effectively. Round-the-clock dosing of the mainstay analgesic rather than PRN dosing maintains stable analgesic blood levels (Pasero et al., 2011).

After round-the-clock administration of pain medication was initiated, R.S.'s behavioral pain score on the PAIN-AD scale decreased to a 2. She was discharged to the SNF, and the hospice staff provided care upon her admission. The hospice team provided the appropriate pain medication orders once she was evaluated. Two weeks after the hospital discharge, the hospice nurse reported that R.S. was moaning and restless, her respiratory rate was 28 breaths per minute, and she was using accessory muscles with each breath. After discussion with R.S.'s daughter, they decided to move R.S. to a local inpatient hospice facility. The nursing staff at the hospice facility attempted to administer the prescribed oral pain medication, but R.S. pocketed the pills in her cheeks and refused to swallow them.

Considering R.S.'s refusal to swallow, how should R.S.'s pain be treated?

a. Lorazepam 0.5 mg sublingually

b. A fan directed at R.S.'s face

c. Liquid morphine (20 mg per ml concentration) given sublingually

d. Morphine infusion at 2 mg per hour continuous

The correct answer is c. Morphine concentrate given sublingually, though absorbed through the gastrointestinal tract, can be administered to patients who are unable or unwilling to swallow pills (Paice & Fine, 2006). Morphine is a good choice to treat her pain, as it will provide some relief of her dyspnea. Answer a is incorrect because lorazepam should be used with caution in older adults because of the risk of delirium, and lorazepam is not a primary treatment for pain. Answer b is also incorrect. A fan may decrease her sense of breathlessness as it stimulates the trigeminal nerve and may provide symptomatic relief. However, it will not treat her pain. Answer d is incorrect as well. In this situation, an infusion of morphine would not be appropriate (Dudgeon, 2006).

Morphine 20 mg/ml concentrate was prescribed to treat R.S.'s pain and shortness of breath. She received 10 mg sublingually every two hours for pain and air hunger. Her respiratory rate decreased to 18 breaths per minute, and she no longer was using accessory muscles. She was not grimacing; however, she remained restless and had intermittent twitching in her extremities. R.S. was incontinent and her urine output was minimal.

What do these physical assessment findings indicate for R.S.?

a. R.S. has developed terminal delirium.

b. R.S. is receiving too much morphine.

c. R.S. may have developed brain metastasis.

d. R.S. is experiencing myoclonus from opioid metabolites.

The correct answer is d. Morphine undergoes glucuronidation and is broken down into active metabolites in the liver and excreted by the kidneys. These metabolites can accumulate at the end of life as body systems, including the kidneys, begin to fail and patients have less oral intake. Switching to an opioid without active metabolites such as fentanyl may be helpful. The addition of a benzodiazepine may be considered to relieve the neurologic consequences (Morita, Tsunoda, Inoue, & Chihara, 2001).

R.S. experienced intermittent exacerbation of confusion, pain, and respiratory distress but remained semiconscious for most of the day (Morita et al., 2001). Her medication regimen was changed to a 2 mg per hour continuous morphine infusion. Lorazepam 0.5 mg IV was added every four hours for myoclonus. Her respiratory rate was 14 breaths per minute and her nonverbal pain score was 0.

R.S.'s son arrived from out of town for a visit. After seeing his mother, the son became visibly upset and asked to see the nurse. He was angry and asked, "What are you people doing, trying to kill her with this morphine?" How can the nurse best address the son's concerns?

a. Agree with the son's concerns, and ask the physician to decrease the rate.

b. Validate the son's distress, and ask him to tell you more about his concern.

c. Tell the son that morphine does hasten death, but at least his mother is comfortable.

d. Refer the son to his sister, the power of attorney, for more information.

The correct answer is b. Many patients, families, and healthcare providers alike have a belief that morphine hastens death. For example, the risk of respiratory depression is overestimated by many. The use of morphine at the end of life using appropriate dosing guidelines is done with the intent of relieving symptoms, and the potential unintended side effects and adverse effects are minimal. Appropriate pain management, including use of morphine, does not hasten death (Bengoechea, Gutiérrez, Vrotsou, Onaindia, & Lopez, 2010; Vitetta, Kenner, & Sali, 2005; Von Gunten, 2008).

R.S. had not had any oral intake for five days and slipped into a coma. She did not exhibit outward signs of discomfort, such as moaning, grimacing, restlessness, or use of accessory muscles with breathing. The hospice social worker and bereavement counselor spent time working with R.S.'s daughter and son providing education and support. Eight days after admission to the hospice inpatient unit, R.S. began to have irregular breathing with periods of apnea. Her legs and arms became mottled and blotchy appearing. Both of her children were present when R.S. died. With careful attention to symptoms and pain management, R.S.'s symptoms were controlled and her death peaceful.

References

Bengoechea, I., Gutiérrez, S.G., Vrotsou, F., Onaindia, M.J., & Lopez, J.M. (2010). Opioid use at the end of life and survival in a hospital at home unit. *Journal of Palliative Medicine, 13,* 1079–1083. doi:10.1089/jpm.2010.0031

Coyle, N.M., & Derby, S. (2006). Symptom management of pain. In D.G. Cope & A.M. Reb (Eds.), *An evidence-based approach to the treatment and care of the older adult with cancer* (pp. 397–438). Pittsburgh, PA: Oncology Nursing Society.

Dudgeon, D. (2006). Dyspnea, death rattle, and cough. In B. Ferrell & N. Coyle (Eds.), *Textbook of palliative nursing* (2nd ed., pp. 249–264). New York, NY: Oxford University Press.

Herr, K., Coyne, P.J., Key, T., Manworren, R., McCaffery, M., Merkel, S., ... Wild, L. (2006). Pain assessment in the nonverbal patient: Position statement with clinical practice recommendations. *Pain Management Nursing, 7,* 42–52. doi:10.1016/j.pmn.2006.02.003

Huffman, J., & Kunik, M. (2000). Assessment and understanding pain in patients with dementia. *Gerontologist, 40,* 574–581.

McCaffery, M., Herr, K., & Pasero, C. (2011). Assessment tools. In C. Pasero & M. McCaffery (Eds.), *Pain assessment and pharmacologic management* (pp. 49–143). St. Louis, MO: Elsevier Mosby.

Morita, T., Tsunoda, J., Inoue, S., & Chihara, S. (2001). Effects of high dose opioids and sedatives on survival in terminally ill cancer patients. *Journal of Pain and Symptom Management, 21,* 282–289. Retrieved from http://www.jpsmjournal.com/article/S0885-3924(01)00258-5/fulltext

Paice, J.A., & Fine, P.G. (2006). Pain at the end of life. In B. Ferrell & N. Coyle (Eds.), *Textbook of palliative nursing* (2nd ed., pp. 131–154). New York, NY: Oxford University Press.

Pasero, C., Quinn, T.E., Portenoy, R.K., McCaffery, M., & Rizos, A. (2011). Key concepts in analgesic therapy. In C. Pasero & M. McCaffery (Eds.), *Pain assessment and pharmacologic management* (pp. 301–322). St. Louis, MO: Elsevier Mosby.

Vitetta, L., Kenner, D., & Sali, A. (2005). Sedation and analgesia prescribing patterns in terminally ill patients at the end of life. *American Journal of Hospice and Palliative Care, 22*, 465–473.

Von Gunten, C.F. (2008). #008 Morphine and hastened death, 2nd ed. Retrieved from http://www.eperc.mcw.edu/fastfact/ff_08.htm

Jennifer Gentry, ANP, ACHPN, FPCN
Coordinator, Clinical Services
Duke University Hospital Palliative Care Consult Service
Team Leader, Acute Pain Service and Stress Management
Department of Advanced Clinical Practice
Clinical Associate
Duke University School of Nursing
Durham, North Carolina

A 42-Year-Old Woman With Non-Small Cell Lung Cancer

J.S. is a 42-year-old African American woman with a history of non-small cell lung cancer. She was admitted one week ago with intractable back pain and headache. She had been experiencing worsening dyspnea and anxiety related to the progression of her cancer. A positron-emission tomography scan confirmed new metastases to the brain, bone, and liver. Because of her history of multiple chemotherapy regimens and the progression of her disease, she was no longer a candidate for chemotherapy. J.S.'s recent blood and sputum cultures did not demonstrate any active infection, and palliative radiation was offered to assist with symptom control of dyspnea and pain. On admission to the inpatient unit, she was prescribed morphine 15 mg PO TID and hydromorphone 2 mg IV push (IVP) every three hours PRN for severe pain. One week later, J.S. continued to rate her pain as an 8 on a 0–10 numeric rating scale with 0 indicating no pain and 10 indicating the worst pain. She was restless, crying, and difficult to console. In the past 24 hours, she had been tachycardic and tachypenic. Recognizing the complex pain needs of the patient with advanced cancer, the nurse requested a palliative care consult.

The goal of palliative care for J.S. is to
a. Improve the patient's sleep.
b. Provide symptom management and improve her quality of life.
c. Stop all treatments.
d. Achieve a state of sedation and avoid pain.

The correct answer is b. The goals of palliative care are to provide symptom management, to improve quality of life, to provide comfort, and to maintain the patient's dignity. Although palliative care may improve

J.S.'s sleep and may involve some level of sedation, these are not the goals of palliative care; therefore, answers a and d are incorrect. Answer c is incorrect because palliative care is appropriate for patients with advanced cancer and may also be used in addition to continued aggressive curative treatment. Palliative care provides aggressive symptom management. Although aggressive curative treatments are no longer an issue, the patient will still receive interventions for symptom control (Boyle & Fink, 2009; Mahay, 2008; National Consensus Project for Quality Palliative Care, 2009; Paice, 2010; Raphael et al., 2010). All needs (physical, psychosocial, and spiritual) should be addressed in creating the palliative care treatment plan. Strong communication is a crucial component of palliative care (Dahlin, Kelley, Jackson, & Temel, 2010; Raphael et al., 2010; Walker, 2008).

J.S. reported pain that was "everywhere" (not localized) and occurring in more than one site. She reported that the pain was not always the same. Sometimes it was sharp; sometimes it was burning. Because of J.S.'s widespread disease, she was experiencing somatic, visceral, and neuropathic pain. Somatic pain occurred as a result of cutaneous or deep tissue involvement of the cancer. Visceral pain was attributed to direct organ involvement of the cancer. Neuropathic pain was a result of nervous system involvement of the cancer leading to direct injury of the nerve (Hutton, McGee, & Dunbar, 2006; National Comprehensive Cancer Network, 2012; Walker, 2008). Despite a fairly aggressive pain management plan, she continued to experience breakthrough pain.

Patients with advanced cancer may have complex pain. Complex pain may result from
a. Tumor location, nerve involvement, or metastatic spread of disease.

b. Original tumor location, but never present at metastatic sites.

c. Tumor location and medication-related side effects only.

d. Nerve involvement and metastatic spread of disease only.

The correct answer is a. Patients with advanced cancer often have complex pain needs resulting from the tumor location, original site of disease, nerve involvement of the tumor, and metastatic spread of disease (Hutton et al., 2006; Walker, 2008). Answer b is incorrect because pain present at the original tumor site may also be present in metastatic sites. Answer c is incorrect because tumor location and medication-related side effects are not the only reasons for complex pain. Answer d is incorrect because nerve involvement and metastatic spread of disease are not the only reasons for complex pain.

The palliative care nurse practitioner (NP) met with J.S. to identify goals for her care. J.S.'s husband and parents were at the bedside. J.S. was anxious and experiencing severe pain. She continued to rate her pain as a 9 and described it as beginning in her chest and radiating to her back. J.S. stated that she wanted to be comfortable and able to spend quality time with her family.

In the past 24 hours, J.S. received breakthrough medication of hydromorphone 2 mg IVP every three hours in addition to her scheduled oral morphine; she received a total of 45 mg of oral morphine and 16 mg of hydromorphone in the past 24 hours. J.S. had uncontrolled pain with the current pharmacologic regimen. The NP discontinued the oral morphine and prescribed a fentanyl transdermal patch 25 mcg/hour. The NP also adjusted her pain medication regimen to include the following.

• Hydromorphone 2 mg IVP every hour PRN for mild to moderate pain
• Hydromorphone 4 mg IVP every hour PRN for severe pain
• Lorazepam 1 mg IVP every six hours PRN for anxiety
• Dexamethasone 4 mg IVP every six hours

When converting oral opioids to a fentanyl transdermal patch, which of the following conversion methods is used?

a. Calculate the patient's 24-hour morphine dose and determine the initial dose of transdermal fentanyl by dividing the 24-hour morphine dose by 2 (morphine to fentanyl conversion ratio of 2:1).

b. Convert all opioids received in the past 24 hours to oral hydromorphone equivalents and dose reduce total amount by 75%.

c. Calculate the patient's 24-hour morphine dose and determine the initial dose of transdermal fentanyl by dividing the 24-hour morphine dose by 3 (morphine to fentanyl conversion ratio of 3:1).

d. Convert all opioids received in the past 24 hours to IV hydromorphone and dose reduce total amount by 50%.

The correct answer is a. The conversion of opioids from one form to another is based on the total amount of oral morphine equivalent administered in a 24-hour period. The morphine-to-fentanyl conversion ratio is 2:1; every 2 mg of oral morphine per day is equivalent to 1 mcg per hour of transdermal fentanyl (McPherson, 2010; Pasero, Quinn, Portenoy, McCaffery, & Rizos, 2011). The number of mcg per hour of transdermal fentanyl should be about half the number of milligrams of oral morphine per day.

Two days later, J.S. reported her pain as a 6. She continued to have moderate to severe back pain and a headache. She reported minimal improvement in her pain despite aggressive revisions to her pain management plan. She was restless with moderate anxiety. The nurse acknowledged her anxiety and explored J.S.'s concerns about the end of life and asked her about her spiritual beliefs and needs. J.S. stated she would like to see the chaplain.

J.S. asked the nurse: "Why did God let this happen?" The nurse explored J.S.'s spirituality and related concerns. The nurse recognized that the patient with advanced cancer who experiences intractable pain may have
a. Spiritual distress.
b. Medication tolerance.
c. Myoclonus.
d. Addiction.

The correct answer is a. At the end of life, intractable pain may be related to unresolved emotional or spiritual issues. Psychosocial and spiritual distress may lead to exacerbation of pain in the patient with advanced cancer. Depression and anxiety are common in patients with cancer and may worsen as the end of life becomes imminent. Spiritual distress may also occur; fear of dying, grief, and psychosocial and spiritual distress may affect the degree of pain, as well as alter the patient's expression of pain. Answers b, c, and d are incorrect. Development of drug tolerance or presence of unmanageable side effects, such as myoclonus, may indicate the need for rotating to a different opioid. Increasing the opioid dose or frequency may worsen the unmanageable symptoms. Stopping opioids would significantly worsen pain (Boyle & Fink, 2009; Bush, 2009; Hutton et al., 2006; Torvik et al., 2008). Patients with a painful chronic illness may experience uncontrolled pain because of undertreatment. Undertreated pain often leads to a series of behaviors in which the patient is seeking more drug or different drugs to attempt to achieve pain relief, known as pseudoaddiction. Pseudoaddiction may occur from undertreated pain or other causes such as emotional or spiritual distress. Addiction is associated with drug cravings and the patient's behaviors are adversely affected. Physical dependence occurs when the patient's body becomes physiologically adapted to the drug and withdrawal of the drug leads to a withdrawal syndrome.

Tolerance occurs when the patient is no longer achieving pain control with a dose that provided pain control in the past (Lusher, Elander, Bevan, Telfer, & Burton, 2006; Schneider, 2006–2007).

Over the next few days, J.S. became intermittently confused and difficult to arouse. She moaned when touched and became extremely agitated with verbal and tactile stimulation. She had irregular respirations with two to three seconds of apnea. The nurse completed her assessment, noting accessory muscle use with respiratory effort, tachycardia, and mottling with trace edema to J.S.'s bilateral lower extremities. The nurse continued to administer pain medication as ordered, and monitored her face, legs, activity, cries, and consolability (the FLACC scale) to assess level of pain because of the patient's inability to communicate (American Society for Pain Management Nursing, 2011; Merkel, Voepel-Lewis, Shayevitz, & Malviya, 1997).

After intervention by the palliative care team, the family understood that J.S.'s cancer was advanced, and she was actively dying from her disease. The family wished to continue pain medication to keep her comfortable. The nurse explained to the family that J.S. may be sedated as a side effect from the pain medication, but the intent of treatment is to relieve her suffering.

In treating pain for the actively dying patient, the goal is to relieve suffering. It is morally acceptable to continue the administration of pain medication, even in the presence of apnea. The rule guiding this is the

a. Rule of nines.
b. Rule of double effect.
c. Rule of law.
d. Rule of thumb.

The correct answer is b. The rule of double effect is a guiding principle for healthcare professionals to determine if an act is morally acceptable. Using the rule of double effect, the intent of the act determines whether or not the act is moral (Bruce, Hendrix, & Gentry, 2006). Answers a, c, and d are incorrect. The rule of nines is a measurement used to determine the amount of burned body surface area (Knaysi, Crikelair, & Cosman, 1968). The rule of law is a legal mechanism used to apply various legal principles to government decisions (Bingham, 2006). The rule of thumb is a procedural method used in the division of profit in various industries (Schweihs, 2011).

J.S. received an additional 2 mg IVP dose of hydromorphone because of increasing discomfort (Paice, 2010; Walker, 2008). After the administration of additional hydromorphone, J.S. became less agitated and calm. J.S. died peacefully with her family at her bedside later in the evening on the inpatient unit.

In patients with advanced cancer, pain
a. Decreases with the progression of disease.
b. Is not affected by the progression of disease.
c. Increases with the progression of disease and is often undertreated.
d. Is not present in the progression of disease and treatment is not required.

The correct answer is c. Pain in patients with advanced cancer is often undertreated and usually increases with the progression of disease for many reasons. Appropriate pain treatment is critical to provide comfort and improve quality of life. Answers a, b, and d are incorrect because pain does not always increase with progression of disease, but may be present to varying degrees. Pain is often undertreated in advanced illness (Paice, 2010; Walker, 2008).

References

American Society for Pain Management Nursing. (2011). *Pain assessment in the patients unable to self-report: Position statement with clinical practice recommendations.* Retrieved from http://www.aspmn.org/Organization/documents/UPDATED_NonverbalRevision FinalWEB.pdf

Bingham, T. (2006, November). *The rule of law.* Lecture presented at the Sixth Sir David Williams Lecture Series. Retrieved from http://www.cpl.law.cam.ac.uk/Media/THE%20 RULE%20OF%20LAW%202006.pdf

Boyle, D., & Fink, R. (2009). Palliative care and end-of-life care. In B.H. Gobel, S. Triest-Robertson, & W.H. Vogel (Eds.), *Advanced oncology nursing certification review and resource manual* (pp. 707–735). Pittsburgh, PA: Oncology Nursing Society.

Bruce, S., Hendrix, C., & Gentry, J. (2006). Palliative sedation in end-of-life care. *Journal of Hospice and Palliative Nursing, 8,* 320–327.

Bush, N.J. (2009). Psychosocial management. In B.H. Gobel, S. Triest-Robertson, & W.H. Vogel (Eds.), *Advanced oncology nursing certification review and resource manual* (pp. 637–675). Pittsburgh, PA: Oncology Nursing Society.

Dahlin, C.M., Kelley, J.M., Jackson, V.A., & Temel, J.S. (2010). Early palliative care for lung cancer: Improving quality of life and increasing survival. *International Journal of Palliative Nursing, 16,* 420–423.

Hutton, N., McGee, A., & Dunbar, C. (2006). A guide to cancer pain management. *British Journal of Community Nursing, 13,* 464–470.

Knaysi, G., Crikelair, G., & Cosman, B. (1968). The rule of nines: Its history and accuracy. *Plastic and Reconstructive Surgery, 41,* 560–563.

Lusher, J., Elander, J., Bevan, D., Telfer, P., & Burton, B. (2006). Analgesic addiction and pseudoaddiction in painful chronic illness. *Clinical Journal of Pain, 22,* 316–324.

Mahay, H. (2008, September). Pain management: Important goal in treating cancer patients. *Pharmacy Times,* pp. 28–29. Retrieved from http://www.pharmacytimes.com/publications/issue/2008/2008-09/2008-09-8668

McPherson, M. (2010). *Demystifying opioid conversion calculations: A guide for effective dosing.* Bethesda, MD: American Society of Health-System Pharmacists.

Merkel, S.I., Voepel-Lewis, T., Shayevitz, J.R., & Malviya, S. (1997). The FLACC: A behavioral scoring scale for scoring postoperative pain in young children. *Pediatric Nursing, 23,* 293–297.

National Comprehensive Cancer Network. (2012). *NCCN Clinical Practice Guidelines in Oncology: Adult cancer pain* [v.2.2012]. Retrieved from http://www.nccn.org/professionals/physician_gls/pdf/pain.pdf

National Consensus Project for Quality Palliative Care. (2009). *Clinical practice guidelines for quality palliative care* (2nd ed.). Retrieved from http://www.nationalconsensusproject.org/guideline.pdf

Paice, J. (2010). Pain at the end of life. In B. Ferrell & N. Coyle (Eds.), *Oxford textbook of palliative nursing* (3rd ed., pp. 161–183). New York, NY: Oxford University Press.

Pasero, C., Quinn, T.E., Portenoy, R.K., McCaffery, M., & Rizos, A. (2011). Key concepts in analgesic therapy. In C. Pasero & M. McCaffery (Eds.), *Pain assessment and pharmacologic management* (pp. 301–322). St. Louis, MO: Elsevier Mosby.

Raphael, J., Hester, J., Ahmedzai, S., Barrie, J., Farqhuar-Smith, P., Williams, J., … Sparkes, E. (2010). Cancer pain: Part 2: Physical, interventional, and complimentary therapies, management in the community; acute treatment-related and complex cancer pain: A perspective from the British Pain Society endorsed by the UK Association of Palliative Medicine and the Royal College of General Practitioners. *Pain Medicine, 11,* 872–896. doi:10.1111/j.1526-4637.2010.00841.x

Schneider, J. (2006–2007). Opioids, pain management, and addiction. *Pain Practitioner, 16*(4), 17–24. Retrieved from http://www.jenniferschneider.com/articles/PainPractitioner_10_06.html

Schweihs, R. (2011). The rule of law overrules the rule of thumb. *I.P. Litigator, 17*(5), 8–15.

Torvik, K., Hølen, J., Kaasa, S., Kirkevold, Ø., Holtan, A., Kongsgaard, U., & Rustøen, T. (2008). Pain in elderly hospitalized cancer patients with bone metastases in Norway. *International Journal of Palliative Nursing, 14*, 238–245.

Walker, S. (2008). Updates in non-small cell lung cancer. *Clinical Journal of Oncology Nursing, 12*, 587–596. doi:10.1188/08.CJON.587-596

Mary Lawson, RN, FNP-BC, ACHPN
Family Nurse Practitioner, Palliative Care and Oncology
Our Lady of the Lake Regional Medical Center
Baton Rouge, Louisiana

A 46-Year-Old Man With Metastatic Urothelial Cancer

J.B. is a 46-year-old man who developed back and right leg pain after an injury at work. Prior to admission, he was evaluated by a neurosurgeon and underwent a laminectomy and L5–S1 microsurgical decompression with relief of radicular pain in his leg. J.B.'s history is unremarkable except for the laminectomy. He reported experiencing episodes of hematuria, which resolved in a few months, so he did not report these symptoms to his healthcare team. However, the hematuria occurred again two months later, but work obligations at his construction business kept him from seeking medical attention. The hematuria worsened, and J.B. was evaluated in the emergency department and admitted to the inpatient unit at the hospital. Social history revealed a smoking history of one pack per day for 30 years, alcohol usage of five to six beers per night, and a 26-year exposure to benzene related to his construction business.

Upon admission, the consulting urologist ordered a computed tomography scan/IV pyelogram (CT-IVP), which revealed a bladder mass. Additional workup included a bone scan, which revealed abnormalities in the lumbar spine at L3–L4, and a CT of the chest, which revealed bilateral pulmonary nodules. J.B. had a cystoscopy with biopsy, which revealed a stage IV high-grade transitional cell carcinoma. The biopsies of two lung nodules were also consistent with a primary of urothelial cancer. Hence, the urologist performed a transurethral resection of the bladder tumor with mitomycin C instillation. After surgery, J.B. was referred to a medical oncologist, who evaluated the findings and planned to start radiation therapy and chemotherapy with cisplatin and gemcitabine every 28 days for three cycles once he recovered from surgery.

J.B. went home after surgery and was only able to return to work for a few weeks during his first cycle of chemotherapy. After one month of treatment, J.B. called the medical oncologist's office and spoke to the nurse. He reported right-sided back and hip pain rating an 8–9 on a 0–10 numeric rating scale (NRS). The nurse advised the patient to come in to see the medical oncologist immediately for an evaluation of his symptoms.

An important aspect of the pain assessment is choosing an appropriate pain tool. Which scale would be the best choice for the nurse to use for J.B.?
a. Brief Pain Inventory
b. NRS
c. Visual analog scale
d. Wong-Baker FACES

The correct answer is b. The NRS is an excellent choice for use in both the inpatient and outpatient settings, as it is quick and easy to use and provides the patient's self-report of pain. It can also be used to assess pain relief following interventions. Patients are asked to rate their pain on a scale of 0–10 (McCaffery, Herr, & Pasero, 2011). The Brief Pain Inventory elicits the physical, psychosocial, and neurologic symptoms and risk and contributing factors, but asks patients to discuss their pain over the past 24 hours and requires 10–15 minutes to complete (McCaffery et al., 2011). A visual analog scale has adequate reliability and validity, but may be more difficult to understand and complete than other single-item pain ratings (McCaffery et al., 2011). The Wong-Baker FACES can be an excellent choice for children, as they can point to the face that best shows how they feel (McCaffery et al., 2011). It is important for the nurse to remember that pain assessment is multidimensional and includes more than a pain intensity rating scale. Although the adult pain scales are validated for use, selection is often based on provider and patient choice.

The office nurse conducted the pain history and assessment with J.B. He said, "My right hip and lower back are really hurting" and rated the hip pain as a 3–4 and his back pain as a 5 on the NRS. J.B. was tearful and continued to describe the pain as aching and increasing upon movement. The nurse informed the medical oncologist of her assessment findings.

Based upon the assessment, which of the following may be indicated to initially manage J.B.'s pain?
a. Oxycodone 5 mg/acetaminophen 325 mg (Percocet®) one tablet every four hours
b. Acetaminophen 650 mg one tablet every six hours PRN for pain
c. Ibuprofen 200 mg one tablet every six hours PRN for pain
d. Codeine 30 mg one tablet every four hours PRN for pain
The correct answer is a. The three steps of the World Health Organization (WHO) Pain Relief Ladder address different intensities of pain. In clinical practice, the purpose of step 2 is to assist the clinician in selecting an opioid that may be conventionally preferred for the treatment of moderate to severe pain in the patient who is opioid-naïve, or nearly so. One tablet Percocet every four hours is indicated for treatment of mild-to-moderate pain. Mild-to-moderate pain is often treated with oral analgesics in a fixed combination of opioid and nonopioid, usually acetaminophen or sometimes aspirin (Pasero, Quinn, Portenoy, McCaffery, & Rizos, 2011). Options b, c, and d are incorrect, as they are usually indicated for step 1 of the WHO Pain Relief Ladder, which addresses mild pain and use of nonopioids, such as acetaminophen or a nonsteroidal anti-inflammatory drug (NSAID) and the possibility of an adjuvant analgesic (Pasero, Quinn, et al., 2011). Codeine has limited usefulness and analgesia that is inferior to that of ibuprofen (Pasero, Quinn, et al., 2011).

Over the next 24–48 hours, J.B. continued to experience increased pain in his right hip and lower back despite taking his prescribed analgesic regimen, and he called to report his pain to the office nurse. J.B. rated his pain as a 9 on the NRS, and he had more difficulty moving and getting out of bed. The office nurse advised J.B. to come to the office with his wife immediately. Upon assessing J.B., the nurse noted that he had right leg weakness, and J.B. reported urinary urgency. The nurse notified the medical oncologist of the findings and J.B. was medically transported to the hospital emergency department for a workup of suspected spinal cord compression. Immediate magnetic resonance imaging (MRI) of the spine was ordered along with an IV bolus of morphine 2 mg for pain control prior to the MRI. The results of the lumbar MRI revealed progression of bony metastasis at L3–L4 with compression on the cord at L4. The medical oncologist changed J.B.'s opioids to parenteral to manage his increasing level of pain and consulted the pain management team and the radiation oncologist for palliative radiation. IV dexamethasone was ordered and administered immediately to treat edema related to cord compression. At this time, J.B.'s 24-hour total dose of oxycodone 5 mg was 30 mg.

Which of the following best manages exacerbation of pain?
  a. Increasing the dose of oxycodone
  b. Starting an opioid infusion
  c. Administering intramuscular meperidine 100 mg every four hours PRN
  d. Obtaining an order for ibuprofen 200 mg tablets PO every six hours

The correct answer is b. Options for IV opioid infusions are morphine, hydromorphone, or fentanyl. Choice of drug is based upon previous use, allergies, or sensitivities. Opioids are recommended for moderate to severe, acute, and persistent nociceptive pain (Irwin, Brant, & Eaton, 2012). They bind directly to opioid receptors and do not have a ceiling effect (Pasero, Quinn, et al., 2011). The ceiling effect is when a drug reaches its maximum effect, so that increasing the drug dosage does not increase its effectiveness (Pasero, Portenoy, & McCaffery, 2011). Answer a is incorrect because the oral route would not act quickly to alleviate acute severe pain. Answer c is incorrect because intramuscular meperidine is not recommended for practice. Repeated use of meperidine causes the buildup of metabolites; furthermore, intramuscular administration is not recommended, as it is painful and absorption is unreliable (American Pain Society, 2003). NSAIDs are effective for many types of cancer-related pain, especially pain caused by inflammation (bone metastasis, postoperative pain). Unless contraindicated, NSAIDs should be used routinely to manage acute and persistent pain. However, answer d is incorrect because NSAIDs have a ceiling dose effect, which does not allow for continual dose adjustment (Pasero, Portenoy, et al., 2011).

Convert J.B.'s 24-hour dose of oral oxycodone to IV morphine continuous infusion using an equianalgesic table. Which of the following would be J.B.'s new dose?
a. 1 mg/hour
b. 0.625 mg/hour
c. 0.725 mg/hour
d. 2.25 mg/hour

The correct answer is b. Steps to determine the total 24-hour dose of oral oxycodone and transition to parenteral opioid dosing are as follows.

- Multiply the milligrams by the number of doses in a 24-hour period (5 mg × 6 doses = 30 mg/24 hours). Locate the equianalgesic dose of PO oxycodone in the equianalgesic table (20 mg). Determine the number of equianalgesic dose units in the 24-hour dose by dividing the 24-hour dose of PO oxycodone by the equianalgesic dose of PO oxycodone (30 mg/20 mg = 1.5 units).

- Locate the dose of IV morphine in the equianalgesic table (10 mg) that is approximately equal to 20 mg of PO oxycodone. Determine the 24-hour dose of IV morphine by multiplying the equianalgesic dose of IV morphine by the equianalgesic units of PO oxycodone (1.5 units × 10 = 15 mg/24 hours).
- Divide the 24-hour dose of IV morphine by the number of doses to be given each 24 hours (15 mg/24 = 0.625 mg/hour) (Pasero, Quinn, et al., 2011).

J.B. started radiation therapy to the L3–4 spine to treat cord compression and manage his pain. The pain management team evaluated J.B. the next day on consult rounds. At this time, J.B. rated his pain as a 5 on the NRS while receiving morphine continuous infusion. He said he was able to move in bed, but that his pain increased to 8 on the NRS when walking to the bathroom, and he described his pain as "a shooting pain" radiating from his right hip to ankle.

Which of the descriptions that the patient used to describe his pain is consistent with neuropathic pain?
a. Shooting
b. Pressure
c. Aching
d. Cramping

The correct answer is a. Neuropathic pain is often described as burning, shooting, or similar to an electric shock (Polomano, 2010, p. 64). Neuropathic pain results from damage to the peripheral or central nervous system. Clinical manifestations and symptoms include numbness, tingling, weakness, and pain. The pain is characterized by dysesthesia, hyperesthesia, or a shooting or lancinating sensation, resulting from nerve injury or compression (Pasero & Portenoy, 2011, p. 7). The patient is at risk for neuropathic pain as a result of his cord compression and chemotherapy. Up to 90% of patients receiving cisplatin develop chemotherapy-induced peripheral neuropathy (Tipton, 2009).

J.B. was hospitalized for almost one month to facilitate pain management, radiation therapy, and another cycle of chemotherapy. Pregabalin 150 mg PO three times a day was started for his neuropathic pain. During his hospitalization, the palliative care team was consulted to discuss goals of care because of the progressive nature of J.B.'s disease. J.B. was discharged with palliative care at home along with long-acting and breakthrough opioid therapy for management of his pain. J.B. was unable to return to work because of fatigue and pain. J.B.'s appetite had steadily declined, and he rarely moved from his recliner chair. J.B. and his wife had hoped that his disease would be responsive to treatment, but as J.B. continued to decline and with the support of the palliative care team, the couple realized that cure was no longer a realistic goal. The palliative care team coordinated the transfer of care to home hospice, and J.B. was made comfortable until he died two weeks later in his home surrounded by his spouse and family.

References

American Pain Society. (2003). *Principles of analgesic use in the treatment of acute pain and cancer pain* (5th ed.). Glenview, IL: Author.

Irwin, M., Brant, J., & Eaton, L. (2012). *Putting evidence into practice: Improving oncology patient outcomes—Pharmacologic and nonpharmacologic interventions for pain.* Pittsburgh, PA: Oncology Nursing Society.

McCaffery, M., Herr, K., & Pasero, C. (2011). Assessment. In C. Pasero & M. McCaffery (Eds.), *Pain assessment and pharmacologic management* (pp. 13–176). St. Louis, MO: Elsevier Mosby.

Pasero, C., & Portenoy, R.K. (2011). Neurophysiology of pain and analgesia and the pathophysiology of neuropathic pain. In C. Pasero & M. McCaffery (Eds.), *Pain assessment and pharmacologic management* (pp. 1–12). St. Louis, MO: Elsevier Mosby.

Pasero, C., Portenoy, R.K., & McCaffery, M. (2011). Nonopioid analgesics. In C. Pasero & M. McCaffery (Eds.), *Pain assessment and pharmacologic management* (pp. 177–276). St. Louis, MO: Elsevier Mosby.

Pasero, C., Quinn, T.E., Portenoy, R.K., McCaffery, M., & Rizos, A. (2011). Opioid analgesics. In C. Pasero & M. McCaffery (Eds.), *Pain assessment and pharmacologic management* (pp. 277–622). St. Louis, MO: Elsevier Mosby.

Polomano, R.C. (2010). Neurophysiology of pain. In B. St. Marie (Ed.), *Core curriculum for pain management nursing* (2nd ed., pp. 63–90). Dubuque, IA: Kendall Hunt Publishing.

Tipton, J.M. (2009). Peripheral neuropathy. In L.H. Eaton & J.M. Tipton (Eds.), *Putting evidence into practice: Improving oncology patient outcomes* (pp. 235–241). Pittsburgh, PA: Oncology Nursing Society.

Michelle Nelson, RN, CNS, BC
Clinical Nurse Specialist, Pain Management
Sanford USD Medical Center
Sioux Falls, South Dakota

Cynette Wipf, RN, OCN®, BC
Clinical Care Coordinator
Sanford USD Medical Center
Sioux Falls, South Dakota

A 44-Year-Old Woman With Metastatic Cancer Pain

M.J. is a 44-year-old woman with a history of stage III breast cancer who presented to the emergency department (ED) with reports of pain in her shoulders and ribs. The pain had been worsening over the past two weeks. M.J. reported an aching, stabbing, and throbbing pain that was well localized to the upper back, right shoulder, and right rib cage. M.J.'s treatment history included a right mastectomy followed by chemotherapy with doxorubicin and cyclophosphamide. She had completed two cycles and was scheduled for a follow-up appointment with her medical oncologist this week when she presented to the ED with this new onset of pain. The patient had asthma and a history notable for spinal stenosis secondary to a motor vehicle accident that occurred 14 years ago. At home, M.J.'s chronic back pain was controlled with oxycodone extended release 20 mg PO twice daily and oxycodone immediate release 5 mg PO every three to four hours as needed for breakthrough pain.

Cancer pain can be classified as all of the following *except*
a. Somatic.
b. Visceral.
c. Neuropathic.
d. Hormonal.

The correct answer is d. The nociceptive or inflammatory process is activation of pain-sensitive afferent neural pathways in response to injury. It can be somatic pain originating from damage of the bone, joint, muscle, skin, or connective tissue or visceral pain originating from visceral organs such as the gastrointestinal tract and pancreas. Neuropathic pain, like nociceptive pain, is a descriptive term used to refer to pain that is believed to be sustained by a set of mechanisms that is driven by damage to or dysfunction of the peripheral or central nervous system (Pasero & Portenoy, 2011). Hormonal is an incorrect answer because it is not a classification of pain.

The following pharmacologic interventions are recommended for the management of moderate to severe, non-neuropathic pain *except*
a. Nonsteroidal anti-inflammatory drugs (NSAIDs).
b. Corticosteroids.
c. Opioids.
d. Antidepressants.

The correct answer is d. Opioids are recommended for moderate to severe acute and persistent pain (Irwin, Brant, & Eaton, 2012). They bind directly to opioid receptors and do not have a ceiling dose effect. For steady pain, a long-acting opioid should be administered around the clock. For acute or breakthrough pain, adding an immediate-release opioid on an as-needed basis is appropriate. NSAIDs can be used as an adjunct to opioids to help manage pain. Corticosteroids are effective in pain that has an inflammatory component, such as bone pain (Pasero, Polomano, Portenoy, & McCaffery, 2011). Antidepressants can be used for neuropathic pain (Irwin et al., 2012).

In the ED, M.J. was examined by the medical oncologist. A chest x-ray was ordered and revealed lytic changes in the third and fourth ribs. A conventional isotope bone scan using technetium 99m methylene-diphosphonate was indicated and revealed multiple metastatic lesions in the L3–L4 region and right scapula. M.J. reported a dull, deep, aching sensation increasing in severity over the past several weeks. She reported a pain score of 9 out of 10 on a numeric rating scale (NRS) in the right shoulder and upper back region.

Based on the presenting signs and symptoms, this patient is experiencing which type of pain?
a. Neuropathic
b. Metastatic bone
c. Somatic
d. Visceral

The correct answer is b. A "dull, aching" sensation is most characteristic of bone pain. Neuropathic pain is characterized by burning, shock-like, and electrical sensations and is often accompanied by sensory loss and dysesthesia. Visceral nociceptive pain involves injury to the viscera, and patients usually complain of gnawing, cramping, aching, or stabbing pain depending on the location of the injury. Somatic nociceptive pain involves injury to the bone, joints, or muscles. It is often described as aching, stabbing, throbbing, or pressure-like in quality (Portenoy & Dhingra, 2011).

In the ED, the medical oncologist ordered morphine 2.5 mg IV push every three to four hours PRN. M.J. received four doses every three hours, although her pain remained uncontrolled and she continued to report her pain as a 7 on the NRS. In the ED, M.J. requested morphine every 20 minutes to alleviate her pain. To manage her pain, M.J. was started on patient-controlled analgesia (PCA). The IV route is the most efficient when an immediate analgesic effect is required, such as for acute, severe escalating pain. It allows for rapid titration. Methods of IV administration include bolus, continuous infusion (basal rate), and PCA (Pasero, Quinn, Portenoy, McCaffery, & Rizos, 2011).

The PCA order was based on the hourly total of IV morphine M.J. received in the ED. The PCA pump was set to deliver a basal rate of 1.5 mg of morphine hourly via continuous infusion, a demand dose of 1 mg every 10 minutes with a maximum of six doses per hour, and a clinician bolus dose of 5 mg every four hours PRN. M.J. was admitted to the inpatient oncology unit for continued evaluation and pain control. The pain management team was consulted, and lumbosacral magnetic resonance imaging (MRI) and a computed tomography (CT) scan of the chest was ordered. The lumbosacral MRI results were compared to previous studies from her motor vehicle accident in 1998 and no significant changes were apparent beyond those from her spinal stenosis. The CT scan of the chest revealed multiple metastatic lesions in the right lung and second, third, and fourth ribs. After discussion with the patient and her husband about palliative chemotherapy, which the patient declined to pursue, a consult was made with the palliative care team. M.J. and her spouse opted for comfort measures to palliate her symptoms. She was referred to radiation oncology for palliative radiation to the chest and ribs.

After initiation of the PCA, the pain and palliative care teams continued to evaluate M.J. on the inpatient oncology unit. She reported significant improvement in her pain, scoring it as a 4 on the NRS. She reported decreased pressure and aching in her chest and right shoulder. She was able to walk to the bathroom and move her right arm to perform her activities of daily living with no increase in pain.

The palliative care nurse practitioner reevaluated M.J.'s pain the next day, and her pain score was 3 on the NRS. The discharge plan included follow-up with radiation oncology and the palliative care outpatient clinic. In preparation for discharge, the palliative care team converted the parenteral route morphine to oral opioid medication.

What is the most appropriate mode of medication administration to use in chronic pain conditions such as cancer?
a. By mouth
b. Subcutaneous
c. Patient-controlled analgesia
d. Epidural

The correct answer is a. Chronic pain is more convenient to manage with an oral agent; it is the preferred route because of its simplicity, safety, and noninvasive route of administration (Irwin et al., 2012). Switching to another route of administration is common when acute pain subsides (Pasero, Quinn, et al., 2011).

The distribution of her daily morphine intake is as follows.

- Basal: 1.5 mg every hour = 36 mg of morphine daily
- Demand: 1 mg every 10 minutes × 6 = 6 mg in 24 hours
- Clinician doses: Two doses of 5 mg of morphine = 10 mg in 24 hours
- Total dose = 52 mg of parenteral morphine in 24 hours

Using an equianalgesic chart, determine which 24-hour total oral dose of morphine M.J. should receive.

a. 256 mg
b. 100 mg
c. 156 mg
d. 200 mg

The correct answer is c. According to the opioid equianalgesic table, 10 mg of IV morphine is equivalent to 30 mg of PO morphine (Pasero, Quinn, et al., 2011). M.J. was receiving 52 mg of IV morphine in 24 hours.

- Step 1: Determine M.J.'s current total 24-hour dose of morphine by adding the number of times IV morphine was administered in a 24-hour period. Total dose = 52 mg of parenteral morphine in 24 hours.
- Step 2: Locate the equianalgesic dose of morphine by the IV route in the equianalgesic chart (10 mg).
- Step 3: Determine the number of equianalgesic dose units in the 24-hour dose of morphine by dividing the total 24-hour dose (52 mg) by the equianalgesic dose (10 mg). 52/10 = 5.2 dose units.

- Step 4: Locate the equianalgesic dose of PO morphine in the equianalgesic chart. Morphine is 30 mg.
- Step 5: Determine the 24-hour dose of PO morphine that will be required by multiplying the equianalgesic dose of morphine (30 mg) by the equianalgesic dose units (5.2 units).
  30 mg × 5.2 = 156 mg of oral morphine/24 hours.
- Step 6: Determine the number of doses that would be equianalgesic to what M.J. is currently taking by dividing the total 24-hour dose of morphine (156 mg) by the number of doses that may be taken as prescribed within 24 hours (e.g., morphine PO every eight hours = three doses) (Pasero, Quinn, et al., 2011).
  156/3 = 52 mg per dose of oral morphine.

One week later, M.J. had a follow-up appointment at the outpatient clinic and the palliative care nurse practitioner evaluated her. M.J. reported controlled pain with a pain score of 1 on the NRS while taking the oral morphine regimen. Relieving pain with effective therapeutic agents is a crucial part of cancer treatment. M.J.'s pain and quality of life improved, and she continued to attend the outpatient palliative care clinic weekly.

References

Irwin, M., Brant, J., & Eaton, L. (2012). *Putting evidence into practice: Improving oncology patient outcomes—Pharmacologic and nonpharmacologic interventions for pain.* Pittsburgh, PA: Oncology Nursing Society.

Pasero, C., Polomano, R.C., Portenoy, R.K., & McCaffery, M. (2011). Adjuvant analgesics. In C. Pasero & M. McCaffery (Eds.), *Pain assessment and pharmacologic management* (pp. 623–818). St. Louis, MO: Elsevier Mosby.

Pasero, C., & Portenoy, R.K. (2011). Neurophysiology of pain and analgesia and the pathophysiology of neuropathic pain. In C. Pasero & M. McCaffery (Eds.), *Pain assessment and pharmacologic management* (pp. 1–12). St. Louis, MO: Elsevier Mosby.

Pasero, C., Quinn, T.E., Portenoy, R.K., McCaffery, M., & Rizos, A. (2011). Opioid analgesics. In C. Pasero & M. McCaffery (Eds.), *Pain assessment and pharmacologic management* (pp. 277–622). St. Louis, MO: Elsevier Mosby.

Portenoy, R.K., & Dhingra, L.K. (2011). Assessment of cancer pain. *UpToDate*. Retrieved from http://www.uptodate.com

Fabienne Ulysse, DNP, RN
Assistant Professor of Nursing
Long Island University
Brooklyn, New York
Oncology Clinical Coordinator
Lutheran Medical Center
Brooklyn, New York

Michelle Peters, RN, MSN, FNP
Family Nurse Practitioner, Director of Nursing
Neighborhood and Family Health Center
Bronx, New York

A 57-Year-Old Man With Lung Cancer and Pain

M.L. is a 57-year-old Chinese man who was diagnosed eight weeks ago with stage IIIB non-small cell adenocarcinoma of the lung (T3 N3 M0). Since diagnosis, M.L. has received two cycles of carboplatin and paclitaxel. He was ambulatory and able to perform all self-care, but was unable to work, spending approximately 75% of his waking hours out of bed. He napped for approximately three hours in the afternoons because of fatigue (Eastern Cooperative Oncology Group Performance Status 2 on a scale of 0–5). M.L. experienced mild dyspnea, for which he used oxygen via nasal cannula at home as needed.

M.L.'s and his wife's primary language was Chinese. They both spoke limited English. His children, ages 30 and 33, spoke both languages fluently. M.L.'s medical history was significant for osteoarthritis to his proximal and distal metacarpal phalanges, which was diagnosed three years ago by his primary care physician. His past surgical history included an appendectomy two years ago. He took ibuprofen 400 mg PRN for osteoarthritis. Allergies included shellfish and penicillin. He lived with his wife of 35 years in their own home after emigrating from China 16 years ago. He had a 40 pack year smoking history and he denied use of alcohol or illicit drugs. His father died of colorectal cancer at the age of 72. His mother was alive at the age of 81 with diabetes and history of a cerebrovascular accident. His brother died of a myocardial infarction at 51 years old, and his sister was alive.

M.L. presented to the outpatient oncology clinic with a new onset of pain in his right scapular area, which began approximately four days ago. He was accompanied by his wife and 30-year-old daughter. With his daughter speaking as an interpreter, the oncology nurse was able to ascertain that the pain was exacerbated by movement and "somewhat relieved" after drinking a Chinese herbal supplement. The nurse noted that M.L. guarded his right arm and visibly winced when he attempted to move it in any direction.

When assessing M.L.'s pain level, the nurse used a 0–10 numeric rating scale (NRS). M.L. currently reported his pain level as a 3; however, the nurse was uncertain that he fully comprehended how the scale was read because of the language barrier.

In order to appropriately assess M.L.'s pain given the language barrier, the nurse should use
a. The Wong-Baker FACES rating scale.
b. A medical interpreter.
c. A visual analog scale.
d. A family member to interpret.

The correct answer is b. Language may be a barrier to effective pain assessment and management when English is not the primary language. Without competent language interpretation, it is not possible to adequately assess pain and to teach pain management principles. Medical interpreters receive specialized training and are fluent in the language of the healthcare provider and the patient. The use of a medical interpreter ensures that accurate information is provided to both the patient and family. The use of family members for interpretation is often discouraged because of differences between generations (Briggs, 2008).

Using tools designed to assess pain in children, such as the Wong-Baker scale, often results in suboptimal pain outcomes in the adult population (Narayan, 2010). Although many numeric and visual analog scales have been translated into different languages, the translations may communicate different meanings, which compromise the scales' validity. For example, Chinese (M.L.'s primary language) is read vertically. If a numeric pain tool translated for a Chinese patient is presented horizontally instead of vertically, the patient may be confused as to how to express his pain level (Briggs, 2008; Narayan, 2010).

M.L. denied headaches, dizziness, syncope, tinnitus, chest pain, palpitations, peripheral edema, abdominal pain, nausea or vomiting, dysphagia, constipation or diarrhea, hematochezia, polyuria, or dysuria. As noted previously, he said that he was experiencing dyspnea with mild exertion and the new onset of pain to the right scapular area. Upon physical examination, the nurse's findings revealed a 57-year-old man who appeared older than his stated age. Vital signs were blood pressure 142/84, respiratory rate 22, heart rate 112 and regular, and temperature 97.6°F orally. His pulse oximetry was 98% on 2 L/minute of oxygen by nasal cannula. His weight was 64.5 kg, and his height was 165 cm.

His head was normocephalic with no evidence of trauma, pupils were equal, round, and reactive to light and accommodation, tympanic membranes were clear, turbinates were pink, mucous membranes were moist, and no lymphadenopathy was present. Lung sounds were diminished to the right lower lobe with dullness to percussion. S1 and S2 heart sounds were normal with no murmurs, rubs, or gallops. Abdomen was soft, with no distention, and positive bowel sounds were noted. Heberden and Bouchard nodes were present on the proximal and distal phalanges. Bilateral pedal pulses were palpable. Motor strength was 3/5 to the right upper extremity and 4/5 to the left upper and bilateral lower extremities. Reflexes were +2 in the bilateral upper and lower extremities.

The nurse ascertained from M.L.'s daughter that M.L. and his family were hesitant to discuss his pain with his medical oncologist, because M.L. was apprehensive about taking "strong pain medication." M.L. believed that the need for pain medication may mean that either his disease has progressed or that he may become addicted to the medication. His daughter was concerned that M.L. was not reporting a higher pain level in the presence of his family for fear of not setting a good example of bravery to them, which is important to men in the Chinese culture. The nurse suspected that M.L.'s pain may not be well controlled and wanted to explore some of the barriers to helping him to effectively manage his pain.

In exploring the barriers to cancer pain management in the Chinese American population, which concern is the most significant barrier for M.L.?

a. Tolerance to pain medication
b. Side effects of the medication
c. Being a "good" patient
d. Costs of medication

The correct answer is a. In a study by Edrington et al. (2009), 50 Chinese Americans with cancer pain completed the following instruments: Brief Pain Inventory, Karnofsky Performance Status scale, Barriers Questionnaire (BQ), Hospital Anxiety and Depression Scale, Suinn-Lew Asian Self-Identity Acculturation Scale, and a demographic questionnaire. Perceived barriers to cancer pain were assessed using the BQ scale (in Chinese). The items are rated using 0 (do not agree at all) to 5 (agree very much) Likert scales. The scale consists of nine subscales (fatalism, fear of addiction, desire to be a good patient, fear of distracting physicians, fear of disease progression, tolerance, side effects, religious fatalism, and time for dosage of medications). Higher scores indicate higher levels of perceived barriers. The individual barriers with the highest BQ scale included tolerance to pain medicine, time intervals used for dosage of pain medication, disease progression, and addiction. The Chinese American patients in this study had a 31% higher BQ mean score than that of White patients with cancer. Exploration of M.L.'s concerns along with patient education using a medical interpreter on the principles of pain management may help to alleviate or reduce these barriers (Edrington et al., 2009).

In the course of caring for M.L., the nurse reflected on her own cultural beliefs. The nurse was unfamiliar with the Chinese culture and traditional Chinese medicine in which mind, body, spirit, and nature are seen as united and interrelated (Edrington, Miaskowski, Dodd, Wong, & Padilla, 2007). Im, Liu, Kim, and Chee (2008) noted that Asians have a tendency to neglect reporting cancer pain and often postpone seeking help until the pain is unbearable. In Western culture, alternative therapies such as herbal supplements are not viewed as having as much influence on pain management as pharmacologic therapy.

In regard to the oncology nurse's own cultural beliefs about pain, which of the following should she explore?

a. Which of her own beliefs are evidence based
b. Her coworkers' cultural beliefs
c. Her understanding of the role of culture
d. The notion that all people within a culture have the same beliefs

The correct answer is a. Healthcare providers must examine their own cultural beliefs about pain and examine if these beliefs are evidence based. Understanding the role of culture is important, but stereotypes must be avoided so that care may be provided based on the needs of the individual (Briggs, 2008; Narayan, 2010). Healthcare providers who are unaware of or nonresponsive to cultural variations in pain expression, expectations, perception, and response to pain may interpret patients' behavior and need in terms of their own culture (Shavers, Bakos, & Sheppard, 2010).

Most people tend to believe that attitudes and behaviors that match their own are correct, and those that do not are abnormal, incorrect, or inferior (Narayan, 2010). It is important for nurses to avoid this kind of thinking when a patient expresses or manages pain in a way that does not match the nurses' own beliefs or expectations. Providing care that is culturally sensitive and identifying and attending to barriers related to effective communication may help to prevent inequalities in pain management (Briggs, 2008). Chinese patients with cancer often show improvements in physical health, mental health, sense of control, and social support when they incorporate interventions that integrate the mind, body, and spirit (Edrington et al., 2007).

Asian patients also report significantly lower levels of pain but no differences in symptoms than African Americans, Caucasians, and Hispanics on four different pain scales (Shavers et al., 2010).

The results of a bone scan completed on M.L. revealed an osseous lesion to the right scapula suspicious for metastatic disease. Through the medical interpreter, M.L. reported his pain as a 7 on the NRS. Radiation oncology was consulted for palliative radiation therapy. To address M.L.'s pain, the nurse obtained an order from the medical oncologist for sustained-release oxycodone 30 mg to be administered every 12 hours, with short-acting oxycodone every 3 hours PRN for breakthrough pain. The nurse is concerned that the ingredients in the Chinese herbal supplement may have an interaction with the oxycodone.

While providing education to M.L. about his pain medications along with the use of the herbal supplement, the nurse's best action would be to

a. Advise M.L. to stop drinking the herbal supplement.
b. Consult with the oncology pharmacist to determine potential interactions.
c. Advise M.L to continue drinking the herbal supplement.
d. Advise M.L. to alternate the herbal supplement with the pain medication.

The correct answer is b. Incorporating neutral and beneficial cultural practices into patients' pain management plan honors patients' cultural needs and preferences. Respecting cultural norms promotes value and communication, potentially improving pain outcomes. The healthcare provider's role is to educate the patient and family members so that they may make an informed decision (Narayan, 2010).

The dose of M.L.'s oxycodone is 30 mg to be taken every 12 hours. Based on the nurse's knowledge of appropriate dosing for breakthrough medication, the correct dose of oxycodone immediate release would be
a. 25 mg every four hours PRN.
b. 10 mg every three hours PRN.
c. 15 mg every two hours PRN.
d. 20 mg every three hours PRN.

The correct answer is b. The dosage is based on 10%–15% of 60 mg, which is 6–12 mg (National Comprehensive Cancer Network [NCCN], 2012). The recommended breakthrough dose of short-acting oxycodone should be 10%–15% of the 24-hour controlled-release oral dose per NCCN guidelines.

The nurse and the oncology pharmacist were able to ascertain that the herbal supplement that M.L. was taking would have no interaction with the prescribed oxycodone. M.L. and his family were provided with education about his medication regimen. His concerns about the use of pain medication were addressed by the nurse, the oncologist, and the oncology pharmacist. He agreed to take the medication as prescribed.

M.L. returned to the oncology clinic one week later for a follow-up visit. Through the use of a medical interpreter, the nurse was able to ascertain that M.L.'s pain was well controlled. He reported his pain as a 2 on the NRS and was able to perform his activities of daily living on his current medication and herbal supplement regimen.

Both culture and ethnicity play an important part in the experience and expression of pain (Briggs, 2008). By exploring perceived barriers, examining cultural values, and working within a multidisciplinary team that includes a medical interpreter when necessary, healthcare providers can offer patients a culturally acceptable plan of care.

References

Briggs, E. (2008). Cultural perspectives on pain management. *Journal of Perioperative Practice, 18,* 468–471.

Edrington, J., Miaskowski, C., Dodd, M., Wong, C., & Padilla, G. (2007). A review of the literature on the pain experience of Chinese patients with cancer. *Cancer Nursing, 30,* 335–346. doi:10.1097/01.NCC.0000290813.14571.65

Edrington, J., Sun, A., Wong, C., Dodd, M., Padilla, G., Paul, S., & Miaskowski, C. (2009). Barriers to pain management in a community sample of Chinese American patients with cancer. *Journal of Pain and Symptom Management, 37,* 665–675. doi:10.1016/j.jpainsymman.2008.04.014

Im, E.O., Liu, Y., Kim, Y.H., & Chee, W. (2008). Asian American cancer patients' pain experience. *Cancer Nursing, 31,* E17–E23. doi:10.1097/01.NCC.0000305685.59507.9e

Narayan, M.C. (2010). Culture's effects on pain assessment and management: Cultural patterns influence nurses' and their patients' responses to pain. *American Journal of Nursing, 110*(4), 38–47.

National Comprehensive Cancer Network. (2012). *NCCN Clinical Practice Guidelines in Oncology: Adult cancer pain* [v.1.2012]. Retrieved from http://www.nccn.org/professionals/physician_gls/pdf/pain.pdf

Shavers, V., Bakos, A., & Sheppard, V. (2010). Race, ethnicity, and pain among the U.S. adult population. *Journal of Healthcare for the Poor and Underserved, 21,* 177–220. doi:10.1353/hpu.0.0255

Karen Visich, RN, MSN, ANP-BC, AOCNP®
Palliative Care Nurse Practitioner/Program Coordinator
Robert Wood Johnson University Hospital
Hamilton, New Jersey

A 71-Year-Old Woman With Metastatic Lung Carcinoma

A.F. is a 71-year-old White woman who presents with newly diagnosed stage IV non-small cell lung cancer. A.F. reported a nine-month history of vague chest, left shoulder, and left rib pain and was initially treated by her primary care physician for rheumatoid arthritis with methotrexate and prednisone.

When she achieved no pain relief, the primary care physician ordered a plain x-ray of the left rib. The x-ray showed diffuse osteoporosis and degenerative change of the left rib cage with a nondisplaced fracture involving the anterolateral aspect of the sixth left rib. The primary care physician then ordered a computed tomography (CT) scan of the chest and abdomen. The CT scan showed a 1.7 × 1.4 cm pleural-based lobulated mass, a 2.1 × 1.5 cm left apex mass, and multiple other subcentimeter nodules within the left lower lobe. Several lytic lesions were within the thoracic spine, including T7, T8, T9, T11, a lytic lesion at L3, and a few small lytic lesions involving the left first and second ribs. The primary care physician then ordered a positron-emission tomography (PET) scan. The PET scan revealed innumerable foci of abnormal uptake throughout the visualized skeleton, indicative of metastatic disease, including cervical, thoracic, and lumbar spine, multiple ribs, left scapula, iliac bones, sacrum, and left proximal femur, as well as a fluorodeoxyglucose-avid subpleural pulmonary nodule in the left lower lobe, a pleural mass in the left apex, left pulmonary hilar adenopathy, trace left pleural effusion, and focal activity, right adrenal gland. A CT-guided lung biopsy revealed fragments of malignant cells, consistent with well-differentiated adenocarcinoma. The tumor was positive for thyroid transcription factor-1, consistent with lung cancer. A.F. was referred to a medical oncologist for treatment planning.

A.F.'s oral medications include
- Alprazolam 0.25 mg at bedtime

- Ibuprofen 200 mg BID
- Diazepam 5 mg three times a day

A.F. reported that the pain that was initially across her anterior chest bilaterally changed to a dull pain in her left lower rib area, and she rates the pain as a 9 on a numeric rating scale of 0–10. The pain caused considerable discomfort, especially when she was sitting. Additionally, she was experiencing considerable pain in her left shoulder. She had difficulty moving her arm and lifting objects.

Which of the following validated assessment tools is recommended to assess pain?
a. A visual analog scale
b. The World Health Organization (WHO) Pain Relief Ladder
c. Karnofsky Performance Status Scale
d. Eastern Cooperative Oncology Group Performance Status

The correct answer is a. A visual analog scale is a frequently used standardized scale that facilitates patient self-reported pain assessment (Ripamonti, Bandieri, & Roila, 2011). Answer b is incorrect because the WHO Pain Relief Ladder facilitates pain medication prescribing, and answers c and d are incorrect because these are both performance status scales. Pain assessment should include onset, type, site, duration, intensity, triggers and alleviating factors, use of analgesics and their efficacy and tolerance, functional status, interference of pain with the patient's daily activities, appetite, work and sleep patterns, and the presence of a caregiver.

A.F. was taking ibuprofen 200 mg PO BID. She rated her pain as a 9. She stated that she was afraid of becoming addicted to narcotics, and she was told that those medications could make her constipated. She said that she was unable to find a comfortable position and was having difficulty sleeping at night. The pain also decreased her appetite and she was losing weight. She said, "I am just sick of this constant pain."

Based on your knowledge of ibuprofen, cancer pain, and the pain assessment of A.F., you recognize that A.F.'s pain medication is

a. Appropriate because she was concerned about constipation.
b. Appropriate because she could become addicted with narcotic pain medications.
c. An inappropriate drug for A.F.'s disease.
d. An inappropriate drug for A.F.'s pain.

The correct answer is d. According to the National Comprehensive Cancer Network (NCCN, 2012) guidelines, opioid-naïve patients experiencing severe pain, described as 7–10 on a pain scale, should receive a short-acting opioid with rapid titration to relieve pain. Because A.F. rates her pain as a 9 and has not been on any previous opioid pain medication, she would be an excellent candidate for opioid pain medication. Answers a and b are incorrect because ibuprofen is not appropriate for patients who rate their pain as a 9. When initiating opioid pain medication, administration of a prophylactic bowel regimen is recommended (NCCN, 2012). The oncology nurse should provide A.F. with education regarding a prophylactic bowel regimen and education and support about the need for opioid pain medication for cancer pain to allay A.F.'s fear of addiction. Answer c is incorrect because pain medication should be prescribed according to pain intensity and the patient's subjective report of pain, not based upon the type of disease.

The immediate priority for A.F.'s treatment plan was for pain control. A.F. was prescribed hydromorphone 2 mg PO every three hours as needed for pain. A.F. was also referred to radiation therapy for palliative treatment to assist with pain management. Before A.F. left the clinic, she asked to speak to the nurse. She told you that she would not start a strong pain medication because she did not want to be constipated.

What is the most appropriate response to A.F.?
a. "Hydromorphone does not cause constipation."
b. "Relieving pain is more important than having constipation."
c. "Let's review information about a bowel regimen."
d. "Patients who are older do not experience constipation."

The correct answer is c. A common side effect from opioids is constipation. Patients should be educated about the risk and strategies to prevent and relieve constipation. Patients should be started on a bowel regimen when starting opioid analgesics (NCCN, 2012). Answer a is incorrect because hydromorphone can cause constipation. Answer b is incorrect because prevention and relief of constipation are equally important to pain control and, when opioid pain medications are started, the risk of constipation will also increase. Answer d is incorrect because age-related changes in absorption, including reduced gastric and intestinal motility, can cause prolonged colon transit time, gastrointestinal distress, and a higher risk for opioid-induced constipation in older adults with cancer (Brant, 2010).

A.F. was prescribed external beam radiation to the left apical mass and left rib for palliative pain control and concurrent chemotherapy consisting of carboplatin area under the curve of 2 and paclitaxel 50 mg/m^2 weekly for eight weeks. Bisphosphonate therapy consisting of denosumab 120 mg subcutaneously every four weeks also was ordered.

Bisphosphonate therapy was ordered to manage which of the following for A.F.?

a. Oncologic treatment of the bone metastasis
b. First-line analgesic treatment for her bone pain
c. Adjunct therapy to improve efficacy of radiation therapy
d. Prevention of skeletal-related events with bone metastasis

The correct answer is d. Bisphosphonate therapy is prescribed for patients with bone metastasis to prevent skeletal-related events. Answers a and c are incorrect because bisphosphonate therapy does not treat cancer metastases involving the bone and does not improve efficacy of concomitant radiation therapy. Answer b is incorrect because little evidence exists to indicate the effectiveness of bisphosphonates as first-line treatment for pain control (Yuen, Shelley, Sze, Wilt, & Mason, 2006).

A.F. returned to the clinic for follow-up one week after starting chemotherapy. She stated that she had no side effects from chemotherapy except for feeling fatigued. She was also very happy that she did not have any hair loss. She took one tablet of hydromorphone every three hours and had better pain control. She rated her pain as a 4. She again expressed fear that she would become addicted; however, she said that she was able to rest better and her appetite improved slightly. A.F. stated that constipation was not a problem, and she had a bowel movement daily. A.F.'s blood counts were acceptable, and chemotherapy continued weekly.

A.F. was seen on week 4 of her chemotherapy treatment. She was tolerating treatment but reported that she was starting to experience intermittent tingling in her fingertips. She was able to write and use utensils. A.F. reported that her pain relief is "about the same" with a rating of 4, and she continued with her pain medications every three hours. Her main report of pain was neuropathic in nature, as she described intermittent tingling in her fingertips. Treatment for her neuropathic pain was discussed, but A.F. said that she did not want any more medications. She was instructed to report any worsening of the tingling in her fingers. Chemotherapy as prescribed continued along with radiation therapy. A.F. was seen again two weeks later, and she reported that she had not been doing well for the past four days. She described the numbness and tingling in her fingers and toes as "miserable." She was unable to pick up or hold objects without dropping them. She stated that she could no longer feel the floor when walking and fell several times at home. The pain associated with neuropathy was "excruciating," and she wanted to stop chemotherapy. After a long discussion with the physician regarding further chemotherapy, she decided to finish radiation and have follow-up scans to assess treatment response. The physician prescribed gabapentin 100 mg PO BID for her neuropathic pain. As A.F. gathered her belongings, she began to cry and said, "I know what gabapentin is because my sister took it. Am I going to have seizures now? How much more can I take?"

What is the most appropriate response to A.F. regarding gabapentin?
a. "Patients with lung cancer can get brain metastasis and have seizures."
b. "Gabapentin does help people like your sister who have seizures. However, in your case, it also can be prescribed to help with your type of numbness and pain in your fingers and toes."
c. "You will be able to sleep better with gabapentin."
d. "Gabapentin will help the pain in your chest."

The correct answer is b. Gabapentin is indicated for postherpetic pain and is recommended as an adjunct analgesic for neuropathic pain in patients with cancer (Dworkin et al., 2007; Irwin, Brant, & Eaton, 2012; NCCN, 2012). Answer a is incorrect because A.F. has not been prescribed gabapentin as a prophylaxis for seizures. Answer c is incorrect because gabapentin is not indicated for insomnia. Answer d is incorrect because gabapentin is not indicated for the acute cancer pain that A.F. has been experiencing in her chest.

A.F. returned to the clinic two weeks later, and her neuropathic pain had not improved. She completed radiation therapy and had more pain in her chest, left shoulder, and left rib. The physician instructed A.F. to increase her dose of hydromorphone to 4 mg every three hours as needed for pain. The physician also increased her gabapentin to 100 mg PO three times a day. A.F. was scheduled for PET/CT chest, abdomen, and pelvis studies in one week with follow-up with the physician.

A.F. returned for follow-up of her scan results. The mass in the left apex improved but unfortunately the right adrenal mass was enlarged and the osseous metastases had all worsened. After a discussion with the physician, A.F. decided that she wanted no more treatment, and the physician referred her to hospice. Her neuropathic pain improved on the adjusted dose of gabapentin, and the hydromorphone maintained her pain control at a 4. The cancer care team coordinated pain assessment and management as a cornerstone of end-of-life care while transitioning A.F. to hospice care in the home setting.

A.F.'s husband called four weeks later to say that A.F. died at home. He was thankful for the team's care and felt that her pain was well managed by the hospice team before she died.

References

Brant, J.M. (2010). Practical approaches to pharmacologic management of pain in older adults with cancer. *Oncology Nursing Forum, 37*(Suppl. 1), 17–26. doi:10.1188/10.ONF.S1.17-26

Dworkin, R.H., O'Connor, A.B., Backonja, M., Farrar, J.T., Finnerup, N.B., Jensen, T.S., ... Wallace, M.S. (2007). Pharmacologic management of neuropathic pain: Evidence-based recommendations. *Pain, 132*, 237–251. doi:10.1016/j.pain.2007.08.033

Irwin, M., Brant, J., & Eaton, L. (2012). *Putting evidence into practice: Improving oncology patient outcomes—Pharmacologic and nonpharmacologic interventions for pain.* Pittsburgh, PA: Oncology Nursing Society.

National Comprehensive Cancer Network. (2012). *NCCN Clinical Practice Guidelines in Oncology: Adult cancer pain* [v.2.2012]. Retrieved from http://www.nccn.org/professionals/physician_gls/pdf/pain.pdf

Ripamonti, C.I., Bandieri, E., & Roila, F. (2011). Management of cancer pain: ESMO clinical practice guidelines. *Annals of Oncology, 22*(Suppl. 6), vi69–vi77. doi:10.1093/annonc/mdr390

Yuen, K.K., Shelley, M., Sze, W.M., Wilt, T., & Mason, M.D. (2006). Bisphosphonates for advanced prostate cancer. *Cochrane Database of Systematic Reviews, 2006*(4). doi:10.1002/14651858.CD006250

Diane G. Cope, PhD, ARNP-BC, AOCNP®
Oncology Nurse Practitioner
Florida Cancer Specialists and Research Institute
Fort Myers, Florida

A 54-Year-Old Man With Acute Myeloid Leukemia

A.S. is a 54-year-old man of Pacific Islander descent. He is married and has three adult children. He has several brothers and sisters with whom he is very close. In the fall of last year he noticed increased shortness of breath when playing basketball, which he played weekly with friends and family. This dyspnea made him go to his primary care physician, where a complete blood count showed a white blood cell count of 9,000 with more than 50% blasts, hemoglobin 13.3, hematocrit 38.7%, and platelets 113,000. He was diagnosed with acute myeloid leukemia and admitted to the inpatient unit at the hospital under the care of the medical oncologist. He received induction chemotherapy with IV idarubicin for three days and IV cytarabine for seven days (3 + 7 regimen); his day 14 marrow indicated 55% blasts.

During this treatment, A.S. experienced National Cancer Institute Cancer Therapy Evaluation Program (2010) grade 2 mucositis consisting of painful erythema, edema, and ulcers, but eating and swallowing were possible. The patient's pain management at this time would most likely consist of

a. Obtaining an order for a continuous IV opioid with an additional patient-controlled analgesia (PCA) option.
b. Encouraging A.S. to tolerate the pain by rinsing more often with normal saline and avoiding the use of opioids.
c. Determining the need for a topical agent for localized lesions and obtaining an order for oral opioids to facilitate mouth care and oral intake.

d. Obtaining an order for a nonsteroidal anti-inflammatory drug (NSAID) to decrease the inflammation A.S. is experiencing from oral microorganisms.

The correct answer is c. Grade 2 mucositis does not typically require IV opioid intervention. Pain control must be addressed proactively and should most likely be administered routinely around the clock to avoid allowing it to become severe. The intent is to facilitate the ability to do mouth care regularly as well as eat and drink for adequate nutrition. A topical agent would be helpful if A.S. has several separate lesions causing discomfort. However, topical agents alone most likely will not be adequate. Answer a is incorrect because this provides more medication than is usually necessary for grade 2 mucositis; answer b is incorrect because normal saline does not provide pain relief, and oral opioids are the appropriate choice in this instance. Answer d is incorrect because NSAIDs have the potential to decrease platelet aggregation and are unlikely to adequately control his pain (Harris, Eilers, Harriman, Cashavelly, & Maxwell, 2008).

Because of the presence of 55% blasts indicating an incomplete remission, A.S. then received salvage chemotherapy with MEC (mitoxantrone, etoposide, cytarabine), which is indicated for salvage chemotherapy. Only patients younger than 60 years old are typically treated with this regimen for reinduction therapy (Fischer, Knobf, Durivage, & Beaulieu, 2003). He tolerated chemotherapy well, and although his counts were slow to recover, he did not experience any symptoms of mucositis.

A.S. was then discharged from the hospital with a plan to proceed to stem cell transplantation if several criteria were met: his disease was in adequate remission, an appropriate donor was identified, organ function tests were within acceptable ranges, and dental extractions occurred. A bone marrow biopsy in December demonstrated less than 10% cellularity with multilineage hypoplasia. This indicated an adequate remission to proceed to stem cell transplantation.

A.S.'s siblings were not human leukocyte antigen–identical. However, a potential unrelated donor was identified from the donor pool. The donor was a 28-year-old man, O positive, and cytomegalovirus negative. A.S.'s past medical and surgical history is unremarkable except for hypertension and hepatitis as a young child. His social history is significant for alcohol abuse; however, he has been in recovery for more than 10 years. He also has a 30 pack year smoking history. Family history is not significant for cancer.

When the transplantation requirements were met, A.S. was admitted to the hospital for a matched, unrelated donor peripheral stem cell transplant. He received fludarabine and melphalan for his conditioning chemotherapy. His family was supportive and involved with his care. His wife was his primary caregiver.

The plan of care for A.S. will be guided by which of the following?

a. Common side effects include nausea and vomiting, mucositis, and diarrhea. Melphalan is regarded as likely to cause mucositis and the related pain; therefore, a PCA should be ordered for the patient on admission.

b. Because A.S. did not have significant mucositis with the prior chemotherapy, he most likely will not experience mucositis or pain with this protocol.

c. Because of the effect of melphalan on the mucosal membranes, cryotherapy can potentially be beneficial to decrease oral mucositis.

d. The majority of interventions for mucositis approach the problem from a treatment perspective; therefore, the nurse should wait and decide what to do if it becomes a problem.

The correct answer is c. Cryotherapy is seen as beneficial with mucotoxic agents with a short half-life that are being infused over a shorter period of time. The cold decreases the circulation to the oral cavity mucous membranes, which in turn decreases the exposure to the mucotoxicity of the melphalan (Harris, Eilers, Cashavelly, Maxwell, & Harriman, 2009). Answer a is incorrect because although patients receiving stem cell conditioning treatment commonly require PCA, it is not instituted until symptoms are severe. Also, this answer omits the cryotherapy option. Answer b is incorrect because despite prior mucositis being a risk factor for developing mucositis, this preparative regimen is highly mucotoxic; therefore, A.S. is still likely to develop it. Answer d is incorrect because limited effective evidence-based interventions for mucositis are available, and we must work to prevent it because of the impact it can have on the patient's treatment experience and symptoms such as pain (Harris et al., 2008).

You are the nurse preparing to administer A.S.'s melphalan. The order is for 140 mg/m²; the dosage is 275 mg IV infused on day 1 within one hour of reconstitution. You teach the patient and family that melphalan is part of A.S.'s conditioning regimen, intended to clear his bone marrow to make way for the transplanted stem cells. You teach the family and patient that during the infusion, he will need to chew ice and popsicles. This will help decrease the severity and duration of mucositis, which in turn should decrease the severity and duration of pain related to lesions in his mouth.

You provide A.S. with ice and popsicles and explain to the family they should call when he needs more during the melphalan administration, but after 10 minutes he tells you he would rather talk on the phone to his brother who just called him from England than continue with the cryotherapy.

As the registered nurse, your discussion with A.S. is guided by the knowledge that
a. 10 minutes of cryotherapy is adequate; this can be anytime during the melphalan infusion.
b. The total time of cryotherapy is more important than that it occur continuously; the patient can restart cryotherapy for 20 minutes later in the day.

c. Cryotherapy is not evidence based; patient preference and need for family support should take preference.

d. Cryotherapy should start prior to the melphalan and continue during the entire infusion to serve as a vasoconstrictor throughout the 30-minute half-life.

The correct answer is d. Melphalan has a short half-life. Cryotherapy during the duration of the infusion provides protection to the mucous membranes of the oral cavity. The hypothermia must be maintained to provide the desired effect (Harris et al., 2009). Answer a is incorrect because 10 minutes of cryotherapy will not provide adequate hypothermia to protect the oral cavity membranes from the mucotoxic effect of the melphalan. Answer b is incorrect because the important timing consideration for cryotherapy is the duration of the infusion and the half-life of the medication. Because melphalan administration time in this protocol is limited, continuous cryotherapy during infusion is realistic as well as evidence based. Answer c is incorrect because evidence indicates cryotherapy is effective for short infusions of agents such as melphalan with a short half-life. Similarly, it is effective for bolus 5-fluorouracil, but not realistic for 24-hour continuous infusions. Ideally, cryotherapy should start prior to the melphalan infusion and continue during the entire infusion because of melphalan's half-life.

At day +4 after transplant, A.S.'s prescribed oral care regimen was oral rinses with normal saline every four hours and cleaning with oral swabs twice a day. He preferred not to use a toothbrush because he noticed some bleeding now that his platelet count was less than 50,000. A.S. used the swabs regularly, but he did not use the oral rinses consistently.

In order to appropriately assess his oral cavity, you should do all of the following *except*

a. Ask A.S. to rate his pain intensity and how his ability to talk, eat, and swallow are being affected.
b. Describe the character of his saliva.
c. Using a flashlight, examine his lips, tongue, and all surfaces of his oral mucosa.
d. Perform the oral assessment every other day.

The correct answer is d. The other options indicate components that are important aspects of adequate oral assessment. Patient rating of pain is essential because oral cavity pain can be intense. A flashlight is needed to allow adequate visualization of changes. The mucous membranes of the throat and esophagus are affected and influence the ability to talk and swallow. Because these areas are not readily observable, the patient needs to be encouraged to report changes in sensation and ability to talk. He is likely to experience salivary changes that should also be reported in terms of visual observation and the patient's report. Oral cavity changes may occur in a matter of hours; thus, it is important to assess his oral cavity on a more frequent basis for early intervention.

The oral assessment indicates A.S.'s mouth is dry but clear of lesions. He reports some discomfort with swallowing. The best intervention for A.S. at this time would be to

a. Increase oral rinses to every two hours and ensure regular administration of pain medications.
b. Ask the physician for an order of "magic" mouthwash to keep his mucositis from progressing.
c. Keep the treatment plan the same. Explain to the patient that these symptoms are expected and that if he rinses frequently, he will not have problems.
d. Increase oral assessments to every four hours but avoid any other changes at this time.

The correct answer is a. Oral rinses every two hours will aid in maintaining a clean oral cavity because there is normal sloughing of cells and delayed replacement as a result of the chemotherapy. Adequate pain management is important to facilitate sufficient cleansing of the tissues during oral care and oral intake. Topical agents are not likely to be adequate for swallowing relief. Answer b is incorrect because there are multiple recipes for "magic" mouthwashes that often include alcohol-based ingredients. The evidence is not adequate to support their use for mucositis treatment. Also, topical agents are not likely to be sufficient for swallowing relief. Answer c is incorrect because cleansing and pain relief are important to decrease the severity of problems. Further changes are likely, but the severity can still be limited. Oral rinses are important. Answer d is incorrect because A.S.'s oral cavity changes may occur very quickly, and thus assessments should be approximately every two hours while awake and at least every four hours at night.

At day +7 after A.S.'s transplant, his mouth continued to be dry, but his tongue developed pronounced raised red papillae, and he rated his pain on swallowing as severe and as a 7 on the 0–10 numeric rating scale at rest. The pain affected his ability to eat and talk. This concerned his family because in the past A.S. had been rather stoic about his symptoms, and his inability to eat was causing them distress.

At this point, treatment should include all of the following *except*

a. Systemic opioid pain medication on a continuous basis.
b. Continuation of frequent oral rinses and oral swabs.
c. Lip lubricants to prevent drying.
d. Glycerin swabs for cleansing areas of soreness.

The correct answer is d. Glycerin actually causes drying and will contribute to additional oral cavity problems, and thus is not indicated (Harris et al., 2009). Answer a, systemic opioid pain medication on a continuous basis, is appropriate care. At this point, the pain is significant and requires round-the-clock pain medication administration. The opioid of choice may vary from institution to institution. A.S. will also benefit from having additional doses available prior to mouth care and attempts to eat. Topical medications alone will not provide adequate relief. Answer b, to continue frequent oral rinses and oral swabs, is important for cleansing purposes, as the accumulation of debris will increase the likelihood of infections and further oral cavity problems. Answer c is also true, as lips tend to become dry and are prone to cracking. Keeping them moist promotes comfort and decreases the likelihood of breakdown, which can serve as a portal for infection.

By day +12, A.S.'s mucositis had improved, and he no longer required IV opioids. A.S. was discharged on day +20. At that point, his mucositis was resolved, and he was able to eat and drink adequately and no longer required pain medication. His oral cavity continued to be an area for focused assessment because of his risk for graft-versus-host disease. Although his mouth will not totally recover for some time, he should not have any long-term consequences of mucositis. He will be followed closely for graft-versus-host disease and was instructed to report symptoms promptly.

References

Fischer, D.S., Knobf, M.T., Durivage, H.J, & Beaulieu, N.J. (2003). *The cancer chemotherapy handbook* (6th ed.). Philadelphia, PA: Mosby.

Harris, D.J., Eilers, J.G., Cashavelly, B.J., Maxwell, C.L., & Harriman, A. (2009). ONS PEP resource: Mucositis. In L.H. Eaton & J.M. Tipton (Eds.), *Putting evidence into practice: Improving oncology patient outcomes* (pp. 201–213). Pittsburgh, PA: Oncology Nursing Society.

Harris, D.J., Eilers, J., Harriman, A., Cashavelly, B.J., & Maxwell, C. (2008). Putting evidence into practice: Evidence-based interventions for management of oral mucositis. *Clinical Journal of Oncology Nursing, 12,* 141–152. doi:10.1188/08.CJON.141-152

National Cancer Institute Cancer Therapy Evaluation Program. (2010). *Common terminology criteria for adverse events* [v.4.03]. Retrieved from http://evs.nci.nih.gov/ftp1/CTCAE/ CTCAE_4.03_2010-06-14_QuickReference_8.5x11.pdf

Debra Harris, MSN, RN, OCN®
Nurse Manager
Oregon Health & Science University
Portland, Oregon

June Eilers, PhD, RN
Clinical Nurse Researcher
Formerly of The Nebraska Medical Center
Omaha, Nebraska

A 59-Year-Old Man With Non-Small Cell Lung Cancer and Neuropathic Pain

G.K. is a 59-year-old German man. He presented to his primary care physician with persistent, nonproductive cough, fatigue, and 20-pound weight loss over the past six months. He is a former smoker with an Eastern Cooperative Oncology Group Performance Status of 2. He reported some back pain but denied hemoptysis. G.K. commented, "My wife and I were eating better, trying to increase our exercise by walking in the evenings when I get home from work. I just thought that it was good to lose a few pounds. I was tired, but really busy with work so I did not go to the doctor until the cough was so bad that I had to get something for it." His wife added, "He had back pain that began intermittently and became more constant as it has worsened over the past month. The pain is interfering with work and being part of family events. He has not been able to get up and around easily. It is the pain that finally made him agree to seek medical attention."

G.K. reluctantly admitted that he does not like to talk about his pain and discomfort; he thought it was arthritis or a pulled muscle. When asked to rate his back pain on a 0–10 numeric rating scale (NRS), G.K. said, "I do not know how choosing a number is going to help." After the nurse described how to use the NRS, G.K. stated that his pain rating was a 3 at rest and 6 with movement because of an increased radiating sensation that at times felt like knives in his back. G.K. also had three adult children, two sons and a daughter, with one granddaughter. He was employed full-time prior to the illness and an active member of his parish and community.

All of the following are additional pain assessment components for G.K. *except*

   a. The patient's word for pain
   b. Behavioral pain scale
   c. Quality of the pain
   d. Location
      The correct answer is b. Key components of pain assessment are location, intensity, quality, pattern, precipitating and alleviating factors, pain history, including the patient's own word for pain, medication history, and meaning of the pain (Johnston, 2007; McCaffery, Herr, & Pasero, 2011). The intensity of pain is quantified by a pain intensity scale. A behavioral pain scale is more appropriate for a patient who is unconscious, unresponsive, or cognitively impaired. Because G.K. is awake, alert, and oriented, the patient's self-report is the most reliable indicator of his pain (American Pain Society [APS], 2008; McCaffery et al., 2011), making answer b the exception.

      If the patient has difficulty with the pain NRS after the purpose and components have been described, the oncology nurse should
   a. Ask the patient to practice by rating other types of pain.
   b. Use the Wong-Baker FACES scale.
   c. Switch to an alternative pain scale for this assessment only.
   d. Skip this component of the pain assessment.
      The correct answer is a. After the purpose and the components of the pain assessment are described to the patient, a visual of the pain rating scale and the opportunity to practice by rating pain examples are valuable for patient education (Johnston, 2007). It is critical to discuss how quantifying his pain is beneficial to managing the patient's pain. The Wong-Baker FACES scale is more appropriate for a pediatric population. An alternative pain scale is an option when the patient has challenges with concep-

tualizing the NRS. However, the pain scale must be used consistently. Pain intensity is an important component of pain assessment and reassessment (McCaffery et al., 2011).

Psychosocial assessment components that influence a patient's perception of pain include cultural considerations and

a. Pain history.
b. Medication history.
c. Meaning of the pain.
d. Behavioral pain indicators.

The correct answer is c. Cultural considerations, meaning of the pain, and social support affect the patient's perception of pain and pain management (Johnston, 2007; McCaffery et al., 2011).

The primary care physician ordered a chest x-ray for G.K. that revealed a mass in the right lung. Subsequently, a referral was made to a surgeon, who performed a needle biopsy that confirmed stage IIIB adenocarcinoma non-small cell lung cancer. The surgeon consulted medical and radiation oncologists for treatment planning. A computed tomography scan revealed metastatic disease in the lumbar spine. G.K. began external beam radiation for pain relief and combination cisplatin-based chemotherapy. His wife reported that G.K. had been taking ibuprofen and 5 mg hydrocodone/500 mg acetaminophen (Vicodin®) that was in the medicine cabinet from knee replacement surgery the previous year.

At first, G.K. was only taking one tablet of Vicodin at night. The primary care physician provided a new prescription for Vicodin while he was undergoing the diagnostic workup and evaluation. However, for the past 24–48 hours, he had taken two tablets of Vicodin every six hours around the clock.

Applying principles of pain management, what is an appropriate next step in the pain management plan for this patient?

a. Start with a low-dose opioid and titrate slowly.
b. Treat moderate neuropathic pain with opioids only.
c. Administer a long-acting opioid around the clock along with immediate-release opioids for breakthrough pain.
d. Provide IV pain medication in addition to oral analgesics.

The correct answer is c. Key pharmacologic management principles suggest initiation of opioids for moderate to severe nociceptive pain with immediate-release formulations for 24–48 hours. For persistent pain, administer a long-acting opioid with immediate-release opioid for breakthrough pain as needed (APS, 2008; Irwin, Brant, & Eaton, 2012; Johnston, 2007). Use an equianalgesic dosing chart as a guideline for conversions from immediate- to sustained-release opioids. The guideline to start low and titrate slowly pertains to considerations for older adults but is safe practice for all (AGS Panel on Chronic Pain in Older Adults, 2002). Opioids are not the only medications for the treatment of neuropathic pain. Co-analgesics such as anticonvulsants (e.g., gabapentin) may be effective in the treatment of neuropathic pain (APS, 2008). The oral route is preferred for chronic pain management (APS, 2008).

The medical oncologist revised G.K.'s treatment plan for pain and prescribed 30 mg of oxycodone PO every 12 hours with oxycodone PO 5 mg tablets for breakthrough pain every 3 hours as needed.

To prophylactically manage opioid-induced constipation, which of the following is the *most* appropriate intervention?

a. Start bulk laxatives.
b. Begin a combination of stimulant laxative and stool softener.
c. Initiate prokinetic medications.
d. Begin milk of magnesia as needed.
The correct answer is b. The combination of stimulant laxative and stool softener is recommended when initiating opioid therapy (Bisanz et al., 2009). Bulk laxatives are not recommended in managing opioid-induced constipation because of an increased risk for bowel impaction in patients who are poorly hydrated. Prokinetic medications, such as metoclopramide, may assist intestinal motility but are not sufficient as sole agents to manage opioid-induced constipation.

With G.K.'s second cycle of chemotherapy that included cisplatin and paclitaxel, the medical oncologist prescribed zoledronic acid, a bisphosphonate, 4 mg IV over 15 minutes every three to four weeks to prevent additional bone metastasis and delay skeletal-related events, such as pathologic fracture and spinal cord compression.

Prior to administration of a bisphosphonate, such as zoledronic acid, the oncology nurse will assess G.K. for
a. Low serum creatinine.
b. Fluid volume overload.
c. Adherence to taking iron supplements.
d. Symptoms of osteonecrosis of the jaw.
The correct answer is d. According to Fitch et al. (2009), serum creatinine and hydration status are evaluated prior to each administration of zoledronic acid to assess for renal insufficiency or impairment. To decrease the risk of hypocalcemia, calcium and vitamin D supplementation is recommended. An uncommon adverse reaction of zoledronic acid is osteonecrosis of the jaw. The nurse should assess the patient's oral health

prior to initiating therapy and throughout the course of the therapy.

Within a week of his second cycle of chemotherapy, which included cisplatin and paclitaxel, G.K. called the clinic about the numbness and tingling in his hands and feet, making it difficult to work at the computer or walk long distances. The medical oncologist prescribed gabapentin 100 mg PO three times a day.

What strategy for neuropathic pain management is recommended for practice?

a. Corticosteroids are effective in managing only persistent neuropathic pain.
b. All anticonvulsants are recommended.
c. Two or more coanalgesics should be initiated at the same time.
d. Opioids should be given in combination with antidepressants and anticonvulsants.

The correct answer is d. According to Irwin et al. (2012), the combination of opioids, antidepressants, and anticonvulsants is recommended for practice in managing neuropathic pain. Anticonvulsants are not all similar in their effectiveness and side effect profile. For example, although effective in neuropathic pain, phenytoin has unfavorable side effects, such as confusion and ataxia. When initiating coanalgesics, single agents are preferred to evaluate effectiveness and side effects. Over time, other coanalgesics may be prescribed to obtain optimal pain relief. Corticosteroids are effective in managing acute and persistent nociceptive pain.

The oncology nurse performed a brief pretreatment assessment before G.K.'s third cycle of chemotherapy, which revealed "mild pain," rating it at 3, and reports of mild nausea that was relieved by prochlorperazine. G.K. denied vomiting or diarrhea between chemotherapy cycles. He reports constipation and numbness and tingling in his feet but none in his hands. He appears uncomfortable in the recliner. G.K. states, "My back hurts; sometimes it is difficult to find the right position. I stopped walking with my wife in the evenings. My legs feel weak. Sometimes, I am just not steady on my feet. I only took the gabapentin twice a day because it made me too sleepy."

Given these symptoms, the oncology nurse suspects which of the following?
a. Tumor lysis syndrome
b. Spinal cord compression
c. Pathologic fracture
d. Superior vena cava syndrome

The correct answer is b. Back pain, constipation, urinary retention, numbness, paresthesia, and sensory loss in the lower extremities are common signs of spinal cord compression (Kaplan, 2009). Although taxanes, vinca alkaloids, and cisplatin agents are more likely to cause peripheral neuropathies (Polovich, Whitford, & Olsen, 2009), other sensory and motor deficit symptoms, such as constipation, difficulty walking, unsteady gait, and the patient's description of progression, lead the oncology nurse to suspect spinal cord compression.

G.K. was admitted to the inpatient oncology unit after a magnetic resonance imaging scan revealed a lumbosacral spine tumor. He was treated for spinal cord compression with IV corticosteroids to reduce cord edema and relieve his pain of 7 before initiating urgent radiation therapy. During this hospitalization, desipramine, an antidepressant, was ordered in addition to the gabapentin 100 mg TID to determine if the combination would provide more relief from the residual numbness and tingling now attributed to his chemotherapy.

Desipramine was prescribed as an adjunct medication for neuropathic pain. What is *most* important for the oncology nurse to know about this medication?
a. Desipramine should not cause the patient to experience a change in blood pressure.
b. Desipramine should be given in the morning.
c. Desipramine should be given at bedtime.
d. Desipramine should not be given to patients until after a trial of amitriptyline.

The correct answer is b. Desipramine has the best pharmacokinetic profile and should be given in the daytime because insomnia is a significant side effect (Aiello-Laws et al., 2009; APS, 2008). Of the antidepressants, amitriptyline is the most effective but has the least tolerable side effect profile, including hypotension and sedation. Amitriptyline should be taken at bedtime.

Following the treatment plan of radiation and IV corticosteroids, G.K.'s pain improved to a rating of 2 at discharge, his constipation was resolved while on a prescribed bowel regimen, and he was increasing his strength and conditioning with support from physical and occupational therapy. He was discharged home in the care of his wife and daughter with follow-up with the medical oncologist in the outpatient clinic within two weeks.

References

AGS Panel on Chronic Pain in Older Adults. (2002). The management of pain in older persons. *Journal of the American Geriatrics Society, 50*(Suppl. 6), S205–S224. doi:10.1046/j.1532-5415.50.6s.1.x

Aiello-Laws, L.B., Reynolds, J., Deizer, N., Peterson, M., Ameringer, S.W., & Bakitas, M. (2009). Putting evidence into practice: What are pharmacologic interventions for nociceptive and neuropathic cancer pain in adults? *Clinical Journal of Oncology Nursing, 13,* 649–655. doi:10.1188/09.CJON.649-655

American Pain Society. (2008). *Principles of analgesic use in the treatment of acute pain and cancer pain* (6th ed.). Glenview, IL: Author.

Bisanz, A.K., Woolery, M.J., Lyons, H.F., Gaido, L., Yenulevich, M., & Fulton, S. (2009). ONS PEP resource: Constipation. In L.H. Eaton & J.M. Tipton (Eds.), *Putting evidence into practice: Improving oncology patient outcomes* (pp. 93–104). Pittsburgh, PA: Oncology Nursing Society.

Fitch, M., Maxwell, C., Ryan, C., Lothman, H., Drudge-Coats, L., & Costa, L. (2009). Bone metastases from advanced cancers: Clinical implications and treatment options. *Clinical Journal of Oncology Nursing, 13,* 701–710. doi:10.1188/09.CJON.701-710

Irwin, M., Brant, J., & Eaton, L. (2012). *Putting evidence into practice: Improving oncology patient outcomes—Pharmacologic and nonpharmacologic interventions for pain.* Pittsburgh, PA: Oncology Nursing Society.

Johnston, M.P. (2007). Pain. In M. Langhorne, J. Fulton, & S. Otto (Eds.), *Oncology nursing* (5th ed., pp. 680–693). St. Louis, MO: Elsevier Mosby.

Kaplan, M. (2009). Back pain: Is it spinal cord compression? *Clinical Journal of Oncology Nursing, 13,* 592–595. doi:10.1188/09.CJON.592-595

McCaffery, M., Herr, K., & Pasero, C. (2011). Assessment. In C. Pasero & M. McCaffery (Eds.), *Pain assessment and pharmacologic management* (pp. 13–176). St. Louis, MO: Elsevier Mosby.

Polovich, M., Whitford, J.M., & Olsen, M. (Eds.). (2009). *Chemotherapy and biotherapy guidelines and recommendations for practice* (3rd ed.). Pittsburgh, PA: Oncology Nursing Society.

Mary Pat Johnston, RN, MS, AOCN®
Oncology Clinical Nurse Specialist
ProHealth Care Regional Cancer Center
Waukesha Memorial Hospital
Waukesha, Wisconsin

A 62-Year-Old Woman With Breast Cancer and Neuropathic Pain

M.D. is a 62-year-old woman with recurrent estrogen receptor–positive breast cancer who presented with solitary bone metastasis to L2 three years ago. She presented with a one-month history of progressive lower back pain radiating down her buttock and right leg. She described the pain as most intense at bedtime with excruciating distressing pain radiating down her leg, making it impossible to get comfortable. When asked to use a 0–10 numeric rating scale (NRS), she described nighttime pain as 9, and it was associated with poor sleep, fatigue, and emotional exhaustion. She tried ibuprofen without relief. She was seen urgently for evaluation, which led to a magnetic resonance imaging (MRI) scan of her lumbosacral spine, which revealed bone metastasis at L2. A subsequent computed tomography (CT)-guided biopsy of the lesion at L2 confirmed histology consistent with metastatic breast cancer. Full staging with CT scans revealed bone-only metastases with disease noted in several vertebral bodies. Her pain was managed with oxycodone 10 mg PO every four hours as needed, along with short prednisone burst of 40 mg PO for 3 days, with gradual taper over a total of 10 days. M.D. described the steroid as "like magic"; she found that both her pain control and sense of well-being improved. She was able to sleep more comfortably while taking oxycodone 10 mg at bedtime. She subsequently underwent radiation therapy for palliation of pain and began an aromatase inhibitor, letrozole, and a bisphosphonate. She found that taking oxycodone prior to radiation therapy enabled her to tolerate positioning for treatment.

Today, M.D. was seen in the clinic for evaluation of new severe upper back pain described as located just under her scapula with the sensation of a constricting band across her upper back and chest that she described as "like my bra is too tight." At rest, she had no pain but with movement noted increased pain that was severe at times, rated at a 7. She denied any tingling or numbness in her extremities and had no weakness in her extremities. She denied any bowel or bladder dysfunction. Over the past two days, the pain had increased to a 10 when lying down, and M.D. found it very difficult to move without the pain becoming excruciating. She tried to manage with ibuprofen 600 mg PO three times daily. She was reluctant to take anything stronger because she was sure that she must have just pulled the muscles in her back by carrying a laundry basket.

On examination, she had visible mild kyphosis of the upper thoracic spine with tenderness on palpation overlying T4–T5. Her motor and sensory examination was normal. Deep tendon reflexes were symmetric bilaterally. M.D. was admitted because of clinical suspicion for spinal cord compression and the need for an urgent MRI evaluation. She was given IV morphine 10 mg and dexamethasone 10 mg in the infusion unit while awaiting an inpatient bed and prior to the imaging study for comfort. The MRI of the spine revealed several new vertebral body metastases with a new spinal cord compression at T4. She was seen by neurosurgery and radiation oncology. She declined surgery and decided to manage with radiation therapy and use of a thoracolumbosacral orthosis for comfort and added stability. M.D. required 40 mg daily of IV morphine for adequate pain control. She started on gabapentin 300 mg at bedtime with a plan to titrate every three to four days, if tolerated, to symptom relief or improvement. She continued dexamethasone 4 mg PO QID during her hospital stay with a plan to taper to three times a day on discharge. In preparation for discharge, M.D. was converted to sustained-release morphine.

Which of the following doses of sustained-release morphine should the nurse anticipate needing to achieve the same level of comfort?

a. Extended-release morphine 30 mg PO BID
b. Extended-release morphine 60 mg PO BID
c. Immediate-release morphine (MSIR) 10 mg PO every six hours around the clock
d. MSIR 20 mg PO every four hours PRN

The correct answer is a. To calculate the total morphine dose, IV is 40 mg and equianalgesic dosing is 1 mg IV to 3 mg PO; therefore 3 × 40 = 120 mg. Extended-release morphine is dosed every 12 hours, so the dosage should be 60 mg twice per day. National Comprehensive Cancer Network (NCCN) adult cancer pain guidelines recommend initiating long-acting opioids at 50% of daily requirements, so M.D. would start at 30 mg extended-release morphine tablets every 12 hours, and the nurse would monitor the need for breakthrough dosing. It is important to emphasize reassessment of pain so that appropriate adjustments can be made based on analgesia, side effects, and the patient's optimal level of functioning (NCCN, 2012; Paice & Ferrell, 2011).

Which of the following should the nurse anticipate using for breakthrough pain management?
a. 10 mg oxycodone every four to six hours PRN
b. 40 mg oral morphine solution every hour PRN
c. 15 mg morphine immediate release every hour PRN
d. 5 mg morphine solution every four hours PRN
The correct answer is c. Recommended dosing for breakthrough pain for a patient on chronic opioid dosing with a long-acting opioid is 10%–20% of the total daily dose, given every one to two hours PRN (NCCN, 2012).

Patient teaching includes the prevention of which of the following side effects of opioid therapy?
a. Respiratory depression
b. Constipation
c. Insomnia
d. Headache

The correct answer is b. All patients on opioids should begin a bowel regimen with the initiation of opioids. It is the one side effect for which tolerance does not develop (NCCN, 2012; Paice & Ferrell, 2011). Somnolence, not insomnia, can be associated with opioids, particularly a newly increased dose or overmedication. Guidance for treatment of opioid-related sedation includes careful pain assessment, decreasing the dose by 25% increments (if a pain intensity rating of 4 or less can be maintained), and rotation to an alternative opioid if the patient cannot tolerate dose reduction (NCCN, 2012). Integrating the use of a sedation scale as part of a comprehensive pain assessment can provide important information for the clinical team to best manage and adjust medication.

Despite several courses of chemotherapy, M.D. developed persistent progressive disease with involvement of her liver, lungs, and bones. She presented to the clinic with intractable nausea and new left sixth cranial nerve palsy. An MRI of the brain and spine revealed evidence of leptomeningeal disease. She underwent palliative radiation to the base of skull and whole brain but elected to forgo further chemotherapy and was discharged home with hospice. Her analgesic needs increased dramatically with several episodes of pain crisis that required IV morphine during her hospital stay. Her average daily pain score was a 4–5 and at its worst a 10. She achieved comfort with the addition of dexamethasone and titration of morphine. As she prepared for discharge, she was happy with controlling her pain to 1–3 on the NRS. She was receiving extended-release morphine at 150 mg PO BID with MSIR 30–60 mg PO every four hours PRN for breakthrough pain. She developed some intermittent confusion and delirium, had visible myoclonic jerks with acute exacerbation of her back pain, and developed diffuse pain in both legs. The nurse suspected that she may have hyperalgesia attributable to morphine metabolites (morphine-3-glucuronide) (Paice & Ferrell, 2011). In collaboration with the physician and hospice team, M.D. was converted to methadone.

Which of the following will the nurse consider in rotating to this opioid?
a. It is safe to use the straight conversion to calculate dose.
b. QT prolongation is a clinically significant risk; therefore, methadone should be avoided.
c. There is great variability in pharmacokinetics of methadone in patients with cancer.
d. Methadone is among the most expensive analgesics available for use.

The correct answer is c. M.D. was on a dose of morphine greater than 300 mg daily and the 2012 NCCN clinical practice guidelines recommend using 1 mg methadone for every 12 mg morphine as a starting point with a careful assessment of pain control and side effects (NCCN, 2012). M.D. was taking 300 mg extended-release morphine PO as well as breakthrough doses of 180 mg morphine daily for a total of 480 mg daily. A reasonable starting dose of oral methadone would be 10 mg PO every six hours for a total of 60 mg/day (American Pain Society, 2004). This was reduced by 25%–50% to account for the incomplete cross-tolerance (NCCN, 2012). Her myoclonus improved with the addition of small doses of lorazepam as needed and rotating off morphine to methadone (Paice & Ferrell, 2011).

M.D. tolerated conversion to methadone. However, over the next week she continued to decline and died comfortably at home with hospice surrounded by her family.

References

American Pain Society. (2004). *Guideline for the management of cancer pain in adults and children.* Glenview, IL: Author.

National Comprehensive Cancer Network. (2012). *NCCN Clinical Practice Guidelines in Oncology: Adult cancer pain* [v.1.2012]. Retrieved from http://www.nccn.org/professionals/physician_gls/pdf/pain.pdf

Paice, J.A., & Ferrell, B. (2011). The management of cancer pain. *CA: A Cancer Journal for Clinicians, 61,* 157–182. doi:10.3322/caac.20112

Marybeth Singer, MS, ANP-BC, AOCN®, ACHPN®
Oncology Nurse Practitioner and Patient Program Manager
Cancer Center
Tufts Medical Center
Boston, Massachusetts

Appendix A. Equianalgesic Dose Chart

A Guide to Using Equianalgesic Dose Charts*

- *Equianalgesic* means approximately the same pain relief.
- The equianalgesic chart is a guideline for selecting doses for opioid-naïve patients. Doses and intervals between doses are titrated according to individuals' responses.
- The equianalgesic chart is helpful when switching from one drug to another or switching from one route of administration to another.[1]
- Doses in this equianalgesic chart suggest a ratio for comparing the analgesic effects of one drug to those of another.
- The longer a patient has been receiving an opioid, the more conservative the starting dose of a new opioid should be.

Opioid	Oral (PO) (over ~ 4 h)	Parenteral (IM/SC/IV) (over ~ 4 h)	Onset (min)	Peak (min)	Duration (h)[2]	Half-Life (h)
Mu Agonists						
Morphine	30 mg	10 mg	30–60 (PO) 30–60 (MR)[3] 30–60 (R) 5–10 (IV) 10–20 (SC) 10–20 (IM)	60–90 (PO) 90–180 (MR)[3] 60–90 (R) 15–30 (IV) 30–60 (SC) 30–60 (IM)	3–6 (PO) 8–24 (MR)[3] 4–5 (R) 3–4 (IV)[2,4] 3–4 (SC) 3–4 (IM)	2–4
Codeine	200 mg NR	130 mg	30–60 (PO) 10–20 (SC) 10–20 (IM)	60–90 (PO) ND (SC) 30–60 (IM)	3–4 (PO) 3–4 (SC) 3–4 (IM)	2–4

(Continued on next page)

Appendix A. Equianalgesic Dose Chart (Continued)

Opioid	Oral (PO) (over ~ 4 h)	Parenteral (IM/SC/IV) (over ~ 4 h)	Onset (min)	Peak (min)	Duration (h)[2]	Half-Life (h)
Fentanyl	—	100 mcg IV 100 mcg/h of transdermal fentanyl is approximately equal to 4 mg/h of IV morphine[5]; 1 mcg/h of transdermal fentanyl is approximately equal to 2 mg/24 h of oral morphine[5]	5 (OT)[6] 5 (B)[6] 3–5 (IV) 10–15 (IM) 12–16 h (TD)	15 (OT)[6] 5 (B)[6] 15–30 (IV) 30–60 (IM) 24 h (TD)	2–5 (OT)[6] 2–5 (B)[6] 2 (IV)[2,4] 2–3 (IM) 48–72 (TD)	3–4[7] > 24 (TD)
Hydrocodone (as in Vicodin®, Lortab®)	30 mg[8] NR	—	30–60 (PO)	60–90 (PO)	4–6 (PO)	4
Hydromorphone (Dilaudid®)	7.5 mg	1.5 mg[9]	15–30 (PO) 15–30 (R) 5 (IV) 10–20 (SC) 10–20 (IM)	30–90 (PO) 30–90 (R) 10–20 (IV) 30–90 (SC) 30–90 (IM)	3–4 (PO) 3–4 (R) 3–4 (IV)[2,4] 3–4 (SC) 3–4 (IM)	2–3
Levorphanol (Levo-Dromoran®)	4 mg	2 mg	30–60 (PO) 10 (IV) 10–20 (SC) 10–20 (IM)	60–90 (PO) 15–30 (IV), 4–6 (IV)[1,3] 60–90 (SC) 60–90 (IM)	4–6 (PO) 4–6 (SC) 4–6 (IM)	12–15

(Continued on next page)

Appendix A. Equianalgesic Dose Chart (Continued)

Opioid	Oral (PO) (over ~ 4 h)	Parenteral (IM/SC/IV) (over ~ 4 h)	Onset (min)	Peak (min)	Duration (h)[2]	Half-Life (h)
Meperidine (Demerol®)	300 mg NR	75 mg	30–60 (PO) 5–10 (IV) 10–20 (SC) 10–20 (IM)	60–90 (PO) 10–15 (IV) 15–30 (SC) 15–30 (IM)	2–4 (PO) 2–4 (IV)[2,4] 2–4 (SC) 2–4 (IM)	2–3
Methadone (Dolophine®)	(See Chapter 13, pp. 339–350, and Table 13-8 and Box 13-3 in the original source.)					
Oxycodone (as in Percocet®, Tylox®)	20 mg	—	30–60 (PO) 30–60 (MR)[10] 30–60 (R)	60–90 (PO) 90–180 (MR)[10] 30–60 (R)	3–4 (PO) 8–12 (MR)[10] 3–6 (R)	2–3 4–5 (MR)[10]
Oxymorphone	10 mg (10 mg R)	1 mg	30–45 (PO) 15–30 (R) 5–10 (IV) 10–20 (SC) 10–20 (IM)	30–90 (PO) 60 (MR)[11] 120 (R) 15–30 (IV) ND (SC) 30–90 (IM)	4–6 (PO) 12 (MR)[11] 3–6 (R) 3–4 (IV)[2,4] 3–6 (SC) 3–6 (IM)	7–11 2 (paren-teral)
Propoxyphene[12] (Darvon®)	—	—	30–60 (PO)	60–90 (PO)	4–6 (PO)	6–12

(Continued on next page)

Appendix A. Equianalgesic Dose Chart (Continued)

Opioid	Oral (PO) (over ~ 4 h)	Parenteral (IM/SC/IV) (over ~ 4 h)	Onset (min)	Peak (min)	Duration (h)^2	Half-Life (h)
Agonist-Antagonists						
Buprenophrine[13] (Buprenex®)	—	0.4 mg	5 (SL) / 5 (IV) / 10–20 (IM)	30–60 (SL) / 10–20 (IV) / 30–60 (IM)	3 (SL) / 3–4 (IV)[2,4] / 3–6 (IM)	2–3 / 5–6
Butorphanol[13] (Stadol®)	—	2 mg	5–15 (NS)[14] / 5 (IV) / 10–20 (IM)	60–90 (NS) / 10–20 (IV) / 30–60 (IM)	3 (SL) / 3–4 (IV)[2,4] / 3–6 (IM)	3–4
Dezocine (Dalgan®)	—	10 mg	5 (IV) / 10–20 (IM)	ND (IV) / 30–60 (IM)	3–4 (IV)[2,4] / 3–4 (IM)	2–3
Nalbuphine[13] (Nubain®)	—	10 mg	5 (IV) / < 15 (SC) / < 15 (IM)	10–20 (IV) / ND (SC) / 30–60 (IM)	4–6 (IV)[2,4] / 4–6 (SC) / 4–6 (IM)	5
Pentazocine[13] (Talwin®)	50 mg	30 mg	15–30 (PO) / 5 (IV) / 15–20 (SC) / 15–20 (IM)	60–180 (PO) / 15 (IV) / 60 (SC) / 60 (IM)	3–4 (PO) / 3–4 (IV)[2,4] / 3–4 (SC) / 3–4 (IM)	2–3

(Continued on next page)

Appendix A. Equianalgesic Dose Chart (Continued)

*This table provided equianalgesic doses and pharmacokinetic information about selected opioid drugs.

ATC—around-the-clock; B—buccal mucosa; h—hour; IM—intramuscular; IV—intravenous; MR—oral modified-release; ND—no data; NR—not recommended; NS—nasal spray; OT—oral transmucosal; PO—oral; R—rectal; SC—subcutaneous; SL—sublingual; TD—transdermal

[1]An expert panel was convened for the purpose of establishing a new guideline for opioid rotation and recently proposed a two-step approach (Fine, Portenoy, Ad Hoc Expert Panel on Evidence Review and Guidelines for Opioid Rotation, 2009). The approach presented in the text for calculating the dose of a new opioid can be conceptualized as the panel's Step One, which directs clinicians to calculate the equianalgesic dose of the new opioid based on the equianalgesic table. Step Two suggests that clinicians perform a second assessment of patients to evaluate the current pain severity (perhaps suggesting that the calculated dose be increased or decreased) and to develop strategies for assessing and titrating the dose as well as to determine the need for breakthrough doses and calculate those doses. The specific steps described in the examples in the text reflect the panel's two-step approach (see Fine, Portenoy, Ad Hoc Expert Panel on Evidence Review and Guidelines for Opioid Rotation, 2009).

[2]Duration of analgesia is dose dependent; the higher the dose, usually the longer the duration.

[3]As in, e.g., MS Contin® and Oramorph® (8–12 hours) and Avinza® and Kadian® (12–24 hours).

[4]IV boluses may be used to produce analgesia that lasts nearly as long as IM or SC doses; however, of all routes of administration, IV produces the highest peak concentration of the drug, and the peak concentration is associated with the highest level of toxicity (e.g., sedation). To decrease the peak effect and lower the level of toxicity, IV boluses may be administered more slowly (e.g., 10 mg of morphine over a 15-min period); or smaller doses may be administered more often (e.g., 5 mg of morphine every 1–1.5 hours).

[5]This is the ratio that is used clinically.

[6]The delivery system for transmucosal fentanyl influences potency, e.g., buccal fentanyl is approximately twice as potent as oral transmucosal fentanyl.

[7]At steady state, slow release of fentanyl from storage in tissues can result in a prolonged half-life (e.g., 4–5 times longer).

[8]Equianalgesic data are not available.

[9]The recommendation that 1.5 mg of parenteral hydromorphone is approximately equal to 10 mg of parenteral morphine is based on single-dose studies. With repeated dosing of hydromorphone (as during PCA), it is more likely that 2–3 mg of parenteral hydromorphone is equal to 10 mg of parenteral morphine.

[10]As in, e.g., OxyContin®.

[11]As in Opana® ER.

[12]65–130 mg = approximately 1/5 of all doses listed in this chart.

[13]Used in combination with mu agonist opioids, this drug may reverse analgesia and precipitate withdrawal in opioid-dependent patients.

[14]In opioid-naïve patients who are taking occasional mu agonist opioids, such as hydrocodone or oxycodone, the addition of butorphanol nasal spray may provide additive analgesia. However, in opioid-tolerant patients such as those receiving ATC morphine, the addition of butorphanol nasal spray should be avoided because it may reverse analgesia and precipitate withdrawal.

Appendix B. World Health Organization Pain Relief Ladder

WHO has developed a three-step "ladder" for cancer pain relief.
If pain occurs, there should be prompt oral administration of drugs in the following order: nonopioids (aspirin and paracetamol); then, as necessary, mild opioids (codeine); then strong opioids such as morphine, until the patient is free of pain. To calm fears and anxiety, additional drugs—"adjuvants"—should be used. To maintain freedom from pain, drugs should be given "by the clock," that is every 3–6 hours, rather than "on demand." This three-step approach of administering the right drug in the right dose at the right time is inexpensive and 80%–90% effective. Surgical intervention on appropriate nerves may provide further pain relief if drugs are not wholly effective.

Freedom from Cancer Pain

3 Opioid for moderate to severe pain, +/- Non-opioid +/- Adjuvant

Pain persisting or increasing

2 Opioid for mild to moderate pain, +/- Non-opioid +/- Adjuvant

Pain persisting or increasing

1 Non-opioid +/- Adjuvant